So You Want to be a
Brain Surgeon?

Second edition

Edited by

Chris Ward
Consultant Plastic Surgeon and
Honorary Senior Lecturer in
Medical Ethics, Imperial College
School of Medicine, London

Simon Eccles
Specialist Registrar in
Accident and Emergency Medicine,
North Thames Region, London

With a Foreword by
David J. Weatherall

Illustrations by
Jacky Fleming

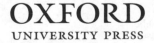

OXFORD
UNIVERSITY PRESS

OXFORD

UNIVERSITY PRESS

Great Clarendon Street, Oxford OX2 6DP

Oxford University Press is a department of the University of Oxford.
It furthers the University's objective of excellence in research, scholarship,
and education by publishing worldwide in

Oxford New York

Auckland Cape Town Dar es Salaam Hong Kong Karachi
Kuala Lumpur Madrid Melbourne Mexico City Nairobi
New Delhi Shanghai Taipei Toronto

With offices in

Argentina Austria Brazil Chile Czech Republic France Greece
Guatemala Hungary Italy Japan South Korea Poland Portugal
Singapore Switzerland Thailand Turkey Ukraine Vietnam

Published in the United States
by Oxford University Press Inc., New York

© Oxford University Press, 2001
Cartoons © Jacky Fleming

The moral rights of the authors have been asserted

Database right Oxford University Press (maker)

First edition published 1997
Reprinted (with corrections) 1998
Second edition published 2001
Reprinted 2001, 2003, 2005, 2006

British Library Cataloguing in Publication Data

Data available

Library of Congress Cataloging in Publication Data

So you want to be a brain surgeon? / edited by Chris Ward, Simon Eccles ; with a
foreword by David J. Weatherall.—2nd ed.
(Oxford medical publications)
Includes bibliographical references and index.
1. Medicine—Vocational guidance. 2. Medical—Vocational guidance—Great Britain.
I. Ward, Chris (Christopher) II. Eccles, Simon. III. Series.
[DNLM: 1. Surgery—Great Britain. 2. Career Choice—Great Britain. 3. Education,
Medical—Great Britain.
WO 21 S675 2001] R690.S6 2001 610.69—dc21 2001016274

ISBN 0 19 263096 2 (Pbk.)

Typeset in Minion by
Footnote Graphics, Warminster, Wiltshire
Printed in Great Britain on acid-free paper by
Biddles Ltd, King's Lynn, Norfolk

Foreword

As I browsed through the contents of this excellent book, pondering on the wonderful diversity of careers open to those with a medical degree and wondering what I would do if I had my time over again, I was reminded of my personal career advice, an episode which lasted all of one minute many years ago. Early in my career I had gone to the United States on a research fellowship and shortly after I returned to Great Britain I had an invitation to return to the States to continue my research. My peers told me that this would be a disastrous move and would surely ruin my career. I therefore plucked up courage and went to seek advice from my first medical chief, Professor Cyril Clarke, later Sir Cyril Clarke and President of the Royal College of Physicians. I briefly outlined the problem. Cyril, a man of few words, was putting the finishing touches to one of his rhesus papers at the time and didn't look up, but after I had finished, simply said "what do you want to do?" "Go back" I said. "Well bugger off then" he replied. Although perhaps rather brief by current career advice standards it was the most valuable 30 seconds of my early career.

Undoubtedly the pressures on medical students and young doctors to develop their careers have increased over the years and begin extremely early. In our misguided education system in this country the decision to become a doctor has to be made by the age of 15 years and I am aghast to hear my colleagues, when interviewing potential medical students, ask which specialty they are going to aim for. I frequently hear groups of students that I am about to talk to on their first day in the clinical school discussing how to manoeuvre their affairs so that they will get on a particular firm as a houseman, a decision that is clearly perceived as likely to make or break their future ambitions. The Calman reforms mean that young doctors must be reasonably sure where they are going within a year or two after qualification, and the Royal Colleges also extract their pound of career-focusing flesh by their rigid training requirements. While undoubtedly much of this is based on admirable intentions, and the realization that the planning of the careers of young doctors in the past has been completely haphazard, there is a genuine danger of stifling originality and the unusual career course as we move into an era of producing doctors by feeding them into this kind of education sausage-machine. The system must allow for the potentially unemployable doctor, or there will be no professors of medicine in the future.

In compiling this excellent compendium of career routes and possibilities for young doctors Christopher Ward & Simon Eccles have done an enormous service to medical students and graduates of the future. I hope that they will buy this book very early on in their careers, browse through it from time to time, and ponder at leisure on the requirements for the richly varied careers that are open to them once they have a basic medical qualification. If they use this book in this way, and the system of postgraduate education that is evolving allows for some flexibility, they will be much better equipped to make appropriate decisions about their careers than many of us were in the past.

A career in medicine can be very lonely, particularly just after qualification and in the early formative years of gaining clinical experience. Although there is an increasing availability of professional career advice much of it is still not very good and certainly is not always given with knowledge of the background and aspirations of the individual to whom it is directed. My advice to medical students and graduates has always been to find themselves a senior mentor who they trust and feel they can go back to discuss their problems and careers over the years. I shall now add the purchase of this book to this simple formula.

D J Weatherall, Oxford

Dedication

To Matt; in the hope that he will discover what he
wants to do and that he will enjoy it.

To Ramanie; now my wife.

Preface to the second edition

The organization and practice of medicine as well as undergraduate and postgraduate education and training have moved on a surprisingly long way in the last four years. The more structured specialist training reforms have been accepted but have substituted different sorts of problems: for example, bottlenecks in the training tube have not been eliminated but relocated. The editors have also moved on. The senior editor is simply older and wiser while the junior partner has progressed to a specialist registrar post in Accident and Emergency Medicine.

As in the first edition we are both grateful for the generosity of so many contributors in providing perceptive and often amusing insights into such a variety of careers. We thank them also for their tolerance of our tailoring of their pieces to fit the style and required page size. We appreciate the suggestions of so many readers who have taken the trouble to contact us. All their ideas have been taken on board and most have been included where possible. Sections have been expanded, notably Working overseas and Psychiatry, and new sections have been added such as Prison healthcare and Occupational medicine. The cartoons of Jacky Fleming have proved to be a great attraction and we thank her for designing more. A few sections were thought to be less relevant to the medical graduate and have been excluded.

At the time of writing it was obvious that the Government intends to introduce further major reforms in the delivery of healthcare which implies that yet another edition may prove necessary, although we hope that it will not be required for several years. Once again we welcome feedback from readers for improvement, future inclusions or modifications in the future.

Finally we thank our families and friends for their support and cajoling as deadlines have come and gone.

London C. W.
January 2001 S. E.

Preface to the first edition

A medical degree offers career opportunities that are unmatched by any other profession. However, the career advice given in medical schools is limited in variety, detail, and scope. Consequently, this book is a collaboration of youth and experience; a student admissions subdean and senior hospital consultant combined with a recently qualified SHO. We hope that this breadth matches the career horizons facing the new medical graduate.

Although we anticipate that medical students and recently qualified doctors will benefit from the description of what is on offer we also expect this book to help potential applicants to medical school in having a clearer idea of what lies ahead and in making the right decision.

In this enterprise we have relied on the expertise of a large number of specialists to provide information with the necessary authority which, as a whole, should be easily accessible to the intended readership. We are enormously indebted to each contributor and gratefully acknowledge their co-operation, professionalism, and patience. We hope that any editorial adjustments will be recognized as a means of keeping within the agreed house style rather than as a personal affront to their writing skills. We are also aware that, within increasing specialization and subspecialization, some may believe that certain topics have been unreasonably excluded. Given the dynamic nature of medicine and its related subjects and the extraneous forces at work on its structure we anticipate that this will not be the only edition of this book and therefore welcome any suggestions for future inclusions, exclusions, or modifications.

We are most grateful to our friends and families who have supported and encouraged us throughout the gestation and labour and, in particular, to Professor Weatherall whose example and wise counsel has been such a strength to so many generations of medical students and graduates.

The publishers and the authors would like to thank Jacky Fleming for the cartoons.

London   C. W.
January 1997   S. E.

Contents

Contributors

1 Introduction

Postgraduate training and Part-time and flexible training
Elizabeth Paice MA FRCP
Dean/Director of Postgraduate
    Medical and Dental Education
    North Thames
University of London
33 Millman Street
London WC1N 3EJ

Medical research
David Evered BSc MD FRCP FIBiol
Whitehall Cottage
Whitehall Lane
Checkendon
Berks RG8 0TR

Women in medicine
Judith Evans MA MBBS FRCSEd
    FRCS
Consultant Plastic Surgeon
Derriford Hospital
Plymouth
Devon W6 8RP

2 Surgery

Breast surgery/surgical oncology
Dudley Sinnett FRCS
Consultant Surgeon
Charing Cross Hospital
Fulham Palace Road
London W6 8RF

Graeme Poston MS FRCS
Consultant Surgeon
The Royal Liverpool University
    Hospital
Prescot Street
Liverpool L7 8PX

Cardiothoracic surgery
Jon Anderson FRCS
Consultant Cardiothoracic Surgeon
Hammersmith Hospital
Du Cane Road
London W12 0HS

Coloproctology and upper gastrointestinal surgery
A J Shorthouse FRCS
Consultant Surgeon
Royal Hallamshire Hospital
Glossop Road
Sheffield S10 2JF

Ear, nose and throat surgery
Grant Bates BSc FRCS
Consultant ENT Surgeon
Radcliffe Infirmary
Woodstock Road
Oxford OX2 6HE

Head and neck surgery
Professor Nicholas Stafford FRCS
Professor in ENT and Head and
    Neck Surgery
The Hull Royal Infirmary
Analaby Road
Hull HU3 2JZ

Maxillofacial surgery
Peter T Blenkinsopp FRCS FDSRCS
Consultant Maxillofacial Surgeon
Queen Mary's Hospital
Roehampton
London SW15 5PN

Plastic and reconstructive surgery
Per Hall FRCS
Department of Plastic and
    Reconstructive Surgery
Addenbrooke's Hospital
Hills Road
Cambridge CB2 2QQ

Hand surgery
David M Evans FRCS
Consultant Plastic Surgeon
The Hand Clinic
Oakley Green
Windsor SL4 4LH

Neurosurgery
Peter Richards FRCS FDSRCS
Consultant Paediatric
    Neurosurgeon
Radcliffe Infirmary
Woodstock Road
Oxford OX2 6HE

Orthopaedic surgery
Andrew J Carr ChM FRCS
Consultant Orthopaedic Surgeon
Nuffield Orthopaedic Centre
Windmill Road
Headington
Oxford OX3 7LD

Trauma surgery
Christopher J K Bulstrode MA
    MCh FRCS(Orth)
Clinical Reader in Orthopaedic
    Surgery
John Radcliffe Hospital
Headington
Oxford OX3 9DU

Paediatric surgery
D M Burge FRCS FRCP
Consultant Paediatric and Neonatal
    Surgeon
Southampton General Hospital
Tremona Road
Southampton SO16 6YD

Transplantation surgery
Paul Lear FRCS
Consultant Vascular and Transplant
    Surgeon
Southmead Hospital
Westbury-on-Trym
Bristol BS10 5NB

Urology
Jonathan Ramsey MS FRCS
Consultant Urologist
Charing Cross Hospital
Fulham Palace Road
London W6 8RF

Vascular surgery
John H N Wolfe MS FRCS
Consultant Vascular Surgeon
St Mary's Hospital
Praed Street
London W2 1NY

3 Reproductive health

Obstetrics and gynaecology

†Professor Michael Hull MD
  FRCOG
Bob Anderson MD FRCOG
Pippa Kyle MD MRCOG
Julian Jenkins DM MRCOG
Department of Obstetrics and
  Gynaecology
St Michael's Hospital
Southwell Street
Bristol BS2 8EG

Phillip Smith FRCOG
Department of Obstetrics and
  Gynaecology
Southmead Hospital
Westbury-on-Trym
Bristol BS10 5NB

Family planning and reproductive healthcare

Tunde Gbolade MRCOG
Fertility Control Unit
St James's University Hospital
Beckett's Street
Leeds LS9 7TF

4 Anaesthetics

Anaesthetics

Raja Jayaweera MA LLB MB BS DA
  FRCA
Consultant Anaesthetist
Whittington Hospital
Highgate Hill
London N19 5NF

Intensive care

David Watson BSc(Hons) FRCA
Consultant and Senior Lecturer in
  Intensive Care Medicine
Barts and the London NHS Trust
West Smithfield
London EC1A 7BE

Simon Eccles MRCS(A&E)Ed
Specialist Registrar in Accident and
  Emergency Medicine
Whittington Hospital
Highgate Hill
London N19 5NF

†(Deceased). Formerly of the
Department of Obstetrics and
Gynaecology, St Michael's Hospital,
Southwell Street, Bristol BS2 8EG.

Pain management

Peter Evans MB BS FRCA
Consultant Anaesthetist
Charing Cross Hospital
Fulham Palace Road
London W6 8RP

5 General practice

General practice

Lyall Eccles MB BS
Orchard Cottage
Loxwood
West Sussex
RH14 0SY

Academic general practice

Professor George K Freeman MD
  FRCGP MRCP
Professor of General Practice
Chelsea and Westminster Hospital
369 Fulham Road

Inner city practice

Brian Hurwitz MRCGP
The Surgery
2 Mitchison Road
London N1 3NG
London SW10 9NH

Remote rural practice

Jon A J Macleod DL FRCGP DCH
  DRCOG
'Tigh-na-Hearradh'
Lochmaddy
Islew of North Uist
Western Isles PA82 5AE

6 General medicine

Audiological medicine

Tony Sirimanna MS FRCS
Consultant Audiological Physician
Great Ormond Street Hospital for
  Children
London WC1N 3JH

Cardiology

William N Hubbard MA FRCP
Consultant Cardiologist
Royal United Hospital
Combe Park
Bath BA1 3NG

Care of the elderly

Stephen G P Webster MA MD
  FRCP
Consultant Physician in Geriatric
  Medicine
Department of Medicine for the
  Elderly
Addenbrooke's NHS Trust
Hills Road
Cambridge CB2 2QQ

Clinical oncology

Barbara Southcott FRCR FFR
Honorary Consultant and Senior
  Lecturer
Department of Radiotherapy and
  Oncology
Charing Cross Hospital
Fulham Palace Road
London W6 8RF

Clinical pharmacology

Professor J M Ritter MA DPhil
  FRCP
Head of Department of Clinical
  Pharmacology
St Thomas's Hospital
Lambeth Palace Road
London SE1 7EH

Dermatology

Jonathan Leonard MD FRCP
Consultant Dermatologist
St Mary's Hospital
Praed Street
London W2 1NY

Endocrinology and diabetes

Philip J Heyburn MD FRCP
Bertram Diabetes Centre
West Norwich Hospital
Brunswich Road
Norwich NR1 3SR

Gastroenterology

B T Cooper MD FRCP
Consultant Physician and
  Gastroenterologist
City Hosital NHS Trust
Dudley Road
Birmingham B18 7QH

Genitourinary medicine

D Daniels MA MRCP
Consultant Physician
Department of Genitourinary
  Medicine
West Middlesex Hospital
Isleworth
Middlesex TW7 6AF

Infectious disease and tropical medicine

Robert N Davidson MD FRCP DTM&H
Consultant Physician and Senior Lecturer
Department of Infection and Tropical Disease
Lister Unit
Northwick Park Hospital
Harrow
Middlesex HA1 3UJ

Medical oncology

Gordon Rustin MD MSc FRCP
Consultant Medical Oncologist
Mount Vernon Hospital
Rickmansworth Road
Northwood
Middlesex HA6 2RN

Nuclear medicine

John Buscombe MD MSc MRCP
Consultant in Nuclear Medicine
Royal Free Hospital
Pond Street
London NW3 2QG

Neurology

Roderick Duncan PhD ChB MRCP
Consultant Neurologist
Institute of Neurological Sciences
Southern General Hospital
Glasgow G51 4TF

Occupational medicine

Ian Lambert MRCGP FFOM
Head of UK Health Services
Shell International Limited
Stanlow Manufacturing Complex
PO Box Ellesmere Port
Cheshire CH65 4HB

Ophthalmology

Nicholas Evans MA DO FRCS FRCOphth
Consultant Ophthalmologist
Royal Eye Infirmary
Aspley Road
Plymouth PL4 6PL

Palliative medicine

Andrew Hoy BSc FRCP FRCR
Medical Director
Princess Alice Hospice
West End Lane
Esher
Surrey KT10 8NA

Renal medicine

Charles Tomson MA DM MRCP
Consultant Nephrologist
Southmead Hospital
Westbury on Trym
Bristol BS10 5NB

Respiratory medicine

Professor A Seed BM PhD FRCP
Department of Respiratory Medicine
Charing Cross Hospital
Fulham Palace Road
London W6 8RF

Public health medicine

Tom W Davies MD MRCP
University Lecturer in Community Medicine
Department of Community Medicine
University Forvie Site
Robinson Way
Cambridge CB2 2SR

Musculosketal medicine

Bryan English MB ChB MRODip(Sports Medicine)
Consultant Physician
Accident and Emergency Department
Royal Hallamshire Hospital
Glossop Road
Sheffield S10 2JF

Rheumatology

Simon Allard MD FRCP
Department of Medicine
West Middlesex Hospital
Isleworth
Middlesex TW7 6AF

Sports medicine

J B King FRCS
Department of Sports Medicine
The London Hospital Medical College
Turner Street
London E1 2AD

Spinal cord injury

David Grundy FRCS
The Duke of Cornwall Spinal Treatment Centre
Salisbury District Hospital
Salisbury SP2 8BJ

7 Accident and emergency medicine

Jonathan Wyatt MB ChB BMed Sci FRCS
Consultant in Accident and Emergency
Royal Cornwall Hospital
Treliske
Truro TR1 3LJ

8 Paediatrics

Christopher Rolles BSc MB ChB MRCP
Consultant Paediatrician
Southampton General Hospital
Tremona Road
Southampton SO16 6YD

9 Diagnostic and interventional radiology

Professor Philip J Robinson FRCP FRCR
Department of Clinical Radiology
St James' Hospital
Leeds LS9 7TF

10 Psychiatry

Child and adolescent psychiatry

Professor David John Cottrell MA MB BS FRCPsych
Professor of Child and Adolescent Psychiatry
Academic Unit of Child and Adolescent Mental Health
School of Medicine
University of Leeds
12A Clarendon Road
Leeds LS2 9NN

Adult psychiatry

Peter Trigwell MB ChB MMedSci MRCPsych
Consultant in Liaison Psychiatry
Leeds General Infirmary
Great George Street
Leeds LS1 3EX

Old-age psychiatry

John David Holmes MA MD MRCP MRCPsych
Senior Lecturer in Liaison Psychiatry of Old Age
Academic Unit of Psychiatry and Behavioural Science
School of Medicine
University of Leeds
15 Hyde Terrace
Leeds LS2 9LT

The psychiatry of learning disability

Tony Holland BSc MB BS MRCP
MRCPsych
University Lecturer in
Developmental Psychiatry
(Learning Disabilities)
Developmental Psychiatry Section
University of Cambridge
Douglas House
18b Trumpington Road
Cambridge CB2 2AH

Psychotherapy

John Hook MSc MRCPsych
Consultant Psychotherapist
Psychological Therapies Service
Department of Psychiatry
Royal South Hants Hospital
Southampton SO14 0YG

Forensic psychiatry

Clive Meux MB BS MRCPsych
Consultant Forensic Psychiatrist,
Oxford Clinic Medium Secure
Unit and Honorary Senior
Lecturer in Forensic Psychiatry,
Institute of Psychiatry, London
Littlemore Mental Health Centre
Sandford Road
Littlemore
Oxon OX4 4XN

11 The Armed Services

The Army

Major Tim J Hodgetts MRCP
FFAEM DipMC RCSEd RAMC
Consultant in Accident and
Emergency Medicine
Frimley Park Hospital
Portsmouth Road
Frimley
Camberley GU16 5UJ

The Royal Air Force

Group Captain M Ranger DAMed
AFOM MRAeS RAF
DDMed Pers, Room G76
Headquarters Personnel and
Training Command
RAF Innsworth
Gloucester GL3 1EZ

Royal Navy

Surgeon Commander John Gabb
Victory Building
HM Naval Base
Portsmouth PO1 3LS

12 Pathology

Chemical pathology

Philip D Mayne MD FRCPI
FRCPath
The Children's Hospital
Temple Street
Dublin 1
Eire

Forensic medicine

Christopher Milroy MD
FRCPath DMJ(Path)
Reader in Forensic Medicine
University of Sheffield
Home Office Pathology
The Medico-legal Centre
Watery Street
Sheffield S3 7ES

Haematology

Professor Sally C Davies FRCP
MRCPath
Regional Director of Research and
Development
NHS Executive
Department of Health
40 Eastbourne Terrace
London W2 3QR

Histopathology and cytopathology

Iain Lindsay MA FRCPath
Consultant Histopathologist
Charing Cross Hospital
Fulham Palace Road
London W6 8RF

Immunology

Jim Darroch MBBS FRCPath
Consultant Immunologist
Royal Liverpool University Hospital
Prescot Street
Liverpool L7 8XP

Medical microbiology

D K Banerjee MD PhD FRCPath
Reader in Medical Microbiology
St George's Hospital Medical
School
Cranmer Terrace
London SW17 0RE

Transfusion medicine

Virge James MA DM FRCPath
MBA
National Blood Service
Longley Lane
Sheffield S5 7JN

Virology

Judy Breuer MD MRCPath
Senior Lecturer in Virology
London Hospital Medical College
37 Ashfield Street
London E1 1BB

13 Biological sciences

Anatomy

Professor John Morris MB BSc MD
Department of Human Anatomy
University of Oxford
South Parks Road
Oxford OX1 3QX

Clinical genetics

Helen Kingston MD FRCP
Consultant Clinical Geneticist
St Mary's Hospital
Hathersage Road
Manchester M13 0JH

Physiology

Frank Harrison BSc PhD
Senior Lecturer in Educational
Development
Imperial College Centre for
Educational Development
Basement, 13 Prince's Gardens
London SW7 1NA

14 Off the beaten track

The Civil Service

Wendy Thorpe MB BS LRCP
MRCS MFPHM
Medical Staffing Officer
Department of Health
Richmond House
79 Whitehall
London SW1A 2NS

Medical management and medical politics

Peter Simpson MA FRCS
MFPHM
Managing Director
Health Management Systems
The White Cottage
21 Clive Road
Esher
Surrey KT10 8PS

Prison healthcare

Roy Burrows MB ChB Dip Pub H
Dip Psyc. Med
Director of Healthcare
Cleland House
Page Street
London SW1P 4LN

Medical research charities

Diana Garnham
General Secretary
Association of Medical Research
29–35 Farringdon Road
London EC1M 3JB

Medical education

Peter McCrorie BSc PhD
Director of Curriculum
Development
St Bartholomew's and The London
School of Medicine and
Dentistry
Queen Mary and Westfield College
Mile End Road
London E1 4NS

Medical ethics

Professor Len Doyal BA MSc
Professor of Medical Ethics
University of London
London Hospital Medical School
Joint Department of Human
Science and Medical Ethics
Turner Street
London E1 2AD

Law

Paul Yates MB BS MRCGP
Senior Legal Adviser—Health Care
Department
St Paul International Insurance Co
Ltd
St Paul House
61–63 London Road
Redhill
Surrey RH1 1NA

Medical defence organizations

Patrick Hoyte MA MRCGP
The Medical Defence Union Ltd
192 Altrincham Road
Manchester M22 4RZ

Medical journalism

David Delvin MB BS MRCGP
c/o A P Watt
20 John Street
London WC1N 2DR

Medical devices

Wynne Weston Davies FRCS
Managing Director
EuroCare (UK) Ltd
Stream Farm
Sedlescombe
East Sussex TN33 0PB

Pharmaceutical physician

Hugh Boardman MA MB ChB
Dip Pharm Med FFPM
6 Stanton Road
Wimbledon SW20 8RL

Complementary medicine

Penny Brougham MB ChB Dip Ac
(Beijing)
The Waldegrave Clinic
82 Waldegrave Road
Teddington
Middlesex TW11 8LG

15 Working overseas

Sallie Nicholas
Head of International Department
British Medical Association
BMA House
Tavistock Square
London WC1H 9JP

Working in overseas aid (International Health Exchange)

Isobel McConnan
Director
International Health Exchange
8/10 Dryden Street
London WC2E 9NA

Christian medical work overseas

Peter Saunders MB FRACS
General Secretary
Christian Medical Fellowship
157 Waterloo Road
London SE1 8XN

Ship's doctor

Gerald Waddington MD ChB
MRCGP
Fleet Medical Advisor
Cunard Line Limited
Mountbatten House
Grosvenor Square
Southampton SO15 2BF

Voluntary Service Overseas

Sue Randall
Press Officer
Voluntary Service Overseas
317 Putney Bridge Road
London SW15 2PN

Working with Médecins Sans Frontières

Jane Ellis MB ChB DTMH MRCP
Médecins Sans Frontières
124/132 Clerkenwell Road
London EC1R 5DJ

Illustrations

The cartoons were drawn by
Jacky Fleming, who holds the
copyright for them.

Terms

The medical hierarchy

Consultant The boss.

Senior registrar Old name, being merged with

Registrar Now called

Specialist registrar The new specialist training grade.

Senior house officer (SHO) The 'lost tribe', to be found doing the donkey work in every hospital in the land.

Junior house officer (HO) Houseplant, housedog, etc.

Other terms in common usage:

Staff grade A non-training grade at SHO/registrar level.

Clinical assistant A non-training grade below consultant, often GPs working in hospitals.

Clinical fellow A non-training grade at registrar level.

Associate specialist Consultant level, but lacks consultant accountability, most commonly found in surgery.

Middle grades Collective name for the above.

Career grades Collective name for all types of training grades.

Non-career grades Collective name for all types of non-training grades.

Preregistration Another term for House officer.

Junior doctor All doctors below consultant level.

Shifts

Full shift Shifts designed to cover the full 24 hours (e.g. accident and emergency department, working flat out but safe in the knowledge you stop when your shift ends).

Partial shift Normal working pattern during the day but including a periodic week of night shifts (e.g. Obstetrics).

Rota system Working 9am–5pm (or 8am–8pm in surgery) during the day then work nights and weekends on-call (i.e. a 1-in-4 or 1-in-5 rota). Fine if quiet but can still result in 56 hours without sleep.

Calman (Report reforms) The current reorganization of training, see Chapter 1.

'Cinderella' specialty A derogatory term for specialties (e.g. family planning, tropical medicine), mainly 9-to-5 with a minimal on-call commitment; tends to be used by those who feel that their specialty is indispensible.

CCST Certificate of Completion of Specialist Training, obtained at the end of training and without which you are not eligible to be a consultant.

Client/Customer Politically correct term and management term for patient, especially common in obstetrics and psychiatry, where it is felt to be less stigmatizing.

Key to summaries

Myth	Those popular myths about each job...
Reality	... and the reality.
Personality	The types of people that do the work.
Best aspects	The best aspects...
Worst aspects	... and worst aspects of the chosen career.
Requirements	Essential and advisable qualifications.

Hours

- 40 hours a week
- 50 hours a week
- 60 hours a week
- 70 hours a week
- >80 hours a week

Numbers — **Total** posts. **Number** of posts a year. **Number** of female consultants as a percentage.

Competitiveness

Stress — The stress of the job, out of 5.

On-calls

- Very rarely disturbed when on-call.
- Occasionally called when on-call.
- Busy when on-call, some sleep possible.
- Very busy, little chance of rest.
- Flat out!

Salary — The **minimum, average,** and **maximum** salary at consultant level. *Note:* The vast majority of practitioners are on the average figure, very few hit the maximum sums, which assume a very considerable private practice.

For further information — Addresses and telephone numbers/fax.

CHAPTER 1

Introduction

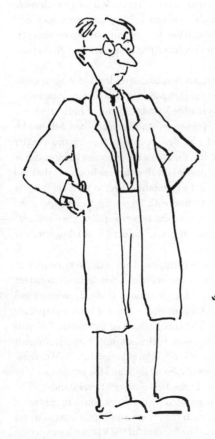

"nerd in a lab coat who can't communicate with patients"... I ask you

A career in medicine remains one of the most popular choices for students of the biological sciences, as judged by the number of applications per place. Guidance and advice for the potential medical student on how to apply and what to expect are easily accessible through books or prospectuses while the universities and medical schools vie to select and seduce the best students by means of open days, lectures, courses and media publicity with lures of the intellectual and material riches that lie ahead and, above all, the job security.

But the reality of life as a medical student has not always matched expectations, even though the educational structure of all medical schools is now light years ahead of what it used to be. Thanks for these changes go to the General Medical Council (GMC) which is responsible for trying to make sure not just that doctors behave themselves and perform to high standards but also that universities teach medical students to the best possible standards. In 1993 the GMC published recommendations for a new format and style of medical undergraduate teaching and learning. Based on a reappraisal of the myriad functions of a doctor, the goals and objectives of teaching were radically revised in order to escape from an overloaded curriculum and the forced feeding and regurgitation of facts in the early science-based years, many of which were of doubtful relevance to life as a doctor. Students are now redirected towards an integrated course involving, among many innovations, exchange and meetings with patients and their families in the first terms of the course, while placing greater emphasis on small group teaching and the facilitation of self-directed learning which more closely matches the enterprise and curiosity of a strongly motivated group of young men and women selected from the top 10% of school leavers. Although the new system may not be perfect it is far more likely to better equip fledgling doctors when they leave the nest even though they are uncertain about which direction to fly.

Next comes the preregistration house officer year which can be soul destroying. Once again intervention was necessary when reports were published about the absurdly long hours, poor supervision and teaching, and unclear training objectives, to which was added a subtle blend of indoctrination. In their concern that all this could undo the good of the revamped student years the GMC implemented a variety of changes through a document called *The New Doctor* so as to ensure a better balance between service commitment and education. But it is the change in specialist training introduced in 1992 that has had the most dramatic impact (see page 6) on all stages leading up to the final appointment at senior level. Inconsistencies, injustices and exploitation had to be eliminated as far as possible while also bringing the training ladder into line with European Union directives. Although the reforms focus mainly on higher specialist training the benefits spilled over into preregistration and senior house officer (SHO) level in terms of better induction, teaching, trainer feedback and supervision, and constructive use of a logbook.

Changes and modifications in teaching and training will continue. That is the very essence of 'being a doctor' and one only has to examine the nature of medicine as a whole to see constant change and evolution in a way that reflects the enterprise and imagination of medical graduates and the changing needs of the society they serve. New specialties continue to emerge while old specialties metamorphose and re-emerge with different names. The composition of the National Health Service (NHS) itself is in continual flux and the style of provision varies not only from government to government but from policy changes within the tenancy of individual governments. Add to these the greater emphasis on continued education, reassessment of clinical skills and the whole notion of professional self-governance and one realizes that the life of a medical graduate never stands still.

Remember that change is more often for the better as recalled by the older editor of this book Chris Ward. He still cringes with embarrassment and shame at the memories of his student days on a medical firm which included a study of venereal diseases. The location of the VD clinic was poorly indicated and found with difficulty. It was in a dimly lit basement of a teaching hospital where 'clinical skills' were learned from examination of the affected parts only, while the top half of the patient was concealed beneath a blanket. Communication skills were not an encouraged ingredient of VD undergraduate teaching where the students were led to believe that what they witnessed was divine retribution for human frailty. Heaven knows what the patients thought of the whole humiliating process, and no student was given the chance to find out. One has only to compare this scenario with the transformation in clinical ambience and philosophy of care taught to students in the redesignated contemporary genitourinary clinics to make one grateful for change.

Nevertheless, even within the more caring and structured environment that has been designed for medical students and recently qualified doctors life can be confusing and disorientating. Few have a clear idea of what they want to do and why they want to do it. Among those who think they know, there are some who regret their decision and change direction; again without making a well informed choice. A few abandon medicine altogether. It is our contention that there would be less regret and disillusion in medicine if doctors had chosen the right career in the first place. But how does one find out?

Some information is given in the later undergraduate years about career options through displays, presentations and designated teaching sessions, but they cannot always be attended by all interested parties. Also, the advice is not comprehensive and tends to be coloured and conditioned by the clinical environment and by the staff and their specialties within the main teaching hospital and the affiliated teaching district general hospitals, which not only fail to represent what is available but may offer prejudiced advice. One still hears the occasional crass view expressed by hospital consultants that general practice is manned by failed doctors, while any thoughts of a career in complementary medicine might be regarded by the odd medical dinosaur to be beyond the pale.

One of the most exciting aspects of medicine is the dazzling number and variety of jobs that should be able to satisfy the appetite of any medical graduate from the traditionalist to the maverick, to the peripatetic and to the more imaginative lateral thinker. There is a glittering display of lights at the end of the tunnel of which every medical student should be made aware. We hope that what follows will help to illuminate the gloom of those students in their final years who may find themselves in the 'lost children' syndrome and to brighten the exhausting and anxious nights and weekends on-call as a preregistration house officer or one of the potentially 'lost tribes' of postregistration SHOs when the mind turns to rest and recreation rather to the patient at hand.

How to use the book

Each main block of career options is introduced by a general career flowchart as illustrated on p. 4 that gives an overview of the training scheme and of the higher qualifications expected until being in a position to apply to consultant level, independent practitioner or equivalent. The specific training requirements to each specialist topic may then be further developed in that particular section while also expanding on the qualities and experience required to step onto the bottom rung. Each contribution then finishes with the description of the scope and opportunities. Facing each main text is an 'at-a-glance' chart that answers the usual questions using symbols rather like those in a Michelin restaurant guide; these are explained on page xviii. However the stress factors and starring of competitiveness and on-calls must be regarded as route guides which are more likely to reflect the perspective of the individual contributors within their particular environment rather than a national perspective. Not all the job options have charts: for example, the section on working overseas

The training ladder from house officer to consultant

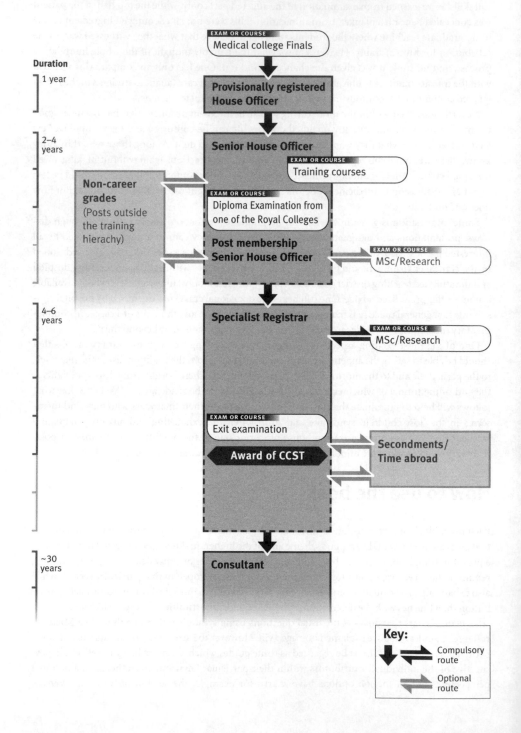

Duration

] 1 year

2–4 years

4–6 years

~30 years

EXAM OR COURSE
Medical college Finals

Provisionally registered House Officer

Senior House Officer

EXAM OR COURSE
Training courses

Non-career grades
(Posts outside the training hierachy)

EXAM OR COURSE
Diploma Examination from one of the Royal Colleges

Post membership Senior House Officer

EXAM OR COURSE
MSc/Research

Specialist Registrar

EXAM OR COURSE
MSc/Research

EXAM OR COURSE
Exit examination

Award of CCST

Secondments/ Time abroad

Consultant

Key:

Compulsory route

Optional route

through the International Health Exchange offers such diversity and flexibility that a summary structure would be inappropriate. The figures on annual expected vacancies or the percentage of women in post change from year to year and it is always worth checking through the relevant 'phone number or website page at the end of each text.

In the wake of the reports on the downside of being a doctor it may be easy to forget what a fulfilling, rewarding, stimulating, exciting and enjoyable profession it can be, providing you choose the right job. Read on and find the right job for you.

What's the money like?

Although the medical course was a long grind and you end up with a massive student overdraft you do at least have the guarantee of a job and the chance not only to pay back the loans but to start accumulating funds for a deposit on a Harley Davidson, a mortgage on a flat or just simply to blow it all on six months' snow-boarding in the Canadian Rockies. So how much will you get paid in the early years of training and beyond?

Before long you will discover that the most widely read medical publication is the classified supplement of the *British Medical Journal* (*BMJ*) which comes out every Friday and in which all the jobs are advertised. There you will also find a page describing the salaries and all the training grades from a first year preregistration houseman at £17 935 a year to the final year of training at £34 930 (correct as of April 2001). These are the basic salary figures, which only apply to a 40-hour week. Overtime is compulsory and paid by a multiplier system, on average this amounts to 1.5 times the basic rate. This added loot comes from supplements negotiated through a new deal for junior doctors which was implemented in December 2000. This deal is a fairly complex banded system based on shifts, on-call rotas and seniority.

It is well worth getting the latest *Junior Doctors' Handbook* from the British Medical Association for an explanation of the pay structure. The book is also invaluable for junior doctors in a host of other information and services such as study and professional leave, maternity leave, accommodation and catering rights, removal and travelling expenses, etc. The main message before you sign the contract for your new job is to make sure that you know precisely the pay and working hours so that you can then agree on fair terms. It is possible in the excitement of being appointed to that job you've always wanted, to commit yourself in writing to what eventually proves to be unreasonable conditions which you will subsequently find are very difficult to negotiate.

In the course of training, it is hoped that through the choices described in this book and your own experience as well as other sources of career advice you will find a job which, in the long term, gives you all the necessary fulfilment. So how much can you expect to get paid once you've achieved your goal?

Through entrepreneurial skills, business acumen and a lot of hard work you can eventually, if you so wish, earn literally millions of pounds a year. Some specialists may opt to work exclusively in private practice and be prepared to compromise any principles they might once have had and, through promotional and advertising patter, persuade the sick and vulnerable to undergo expensive and often inadequate treatment. An obvious example is to be found through cosmetic surgery which is advertised on local radio and in the national tabloids and 'glossies' where the fundamental goal of enhancing the quality of life through safe and well tried procedures may be overwhelmed by the pursuit of money as an end in itself through flashy and hazardous gimmickry.

At the other extreme are those with a greater sense of vocation and altruism who are prepared to make considerable personal sacrifices in order to serve the needs of others. This is summed up in an advertisement for voluntary work abroad: 'Overseas, underpaid .... and the best job in the world'.

However, the majority of medical graduates work within traditional boundaries set by the NHS and universities, which on top of the maximum basic consultant-grade salary of £61 505 (again see the relevant page in the *BMJ* pay scales), allows modest opportunities for private practice and much-deserved icing on the cake.

Depending on how much you contribute to the institution in which you work added money may come in the form of merit awards. On a local level discretionary points are awarded according to your professional performance plus various other activities such as teaching and training, administration and involvement in clinical audit, clinical governance and committee work. You are then personally rewarded according to how many points are aggregated which may be worth up to an additional £12 000 per year. But much larger additional rewards for distinction are made through the National Advisory Committee on Merit Awards. For example, in 1999 481 awards were given of which 37 were A+ worth £60 460 each, 142 A awards at £44 550 and 302 B awards at £25 455 each. There are all sorts of other ways of keeping yourself and your family in style such as insurance reports, acting as a medical expert and delivering invited lectures and articles.

Although General Practitioners (GPs) work in the NHS their pay is governed by a different and complex mechanism described in a book with the long title of *A Statement of Fees and Allowances Payable to General Practitioners in England and Wales* but with a short title of *The Red Book* (Scotland and Northern Ireland have similar arrangements). Income depends on the size, nature and location of the practice and compares very reasonably with the salaries of hospital consultants except for the megabucks available for some of the Harley Street mob or their equivalent outside London.

Providing you don't set your sights too high, with over-extravagant and expensive tastes, or have too many divorces, you will always have the opportunity to earn a comfortable living, to indulge your interests, enjoy good holidays and end up with a secure pension. So just go out there and enjoy it.

Postgraduate training

After five or six years at medical school and successfully completing finals all medical graduates go on to their preregistration year. An increasing number are opting for three jobs of four months each, which gives greater variety than the traditional model of six months in surgery and six in medicine.

The difficult decision comes next. Very few doctors at this stage know exactly what they wish to do for the rest of their careers, so choosing the first SHO post becomes all the more tricky.

The SHO years

The wide variety of choices available are illustrated later in this book but the initial choice can be brought down to: general practice, hospital specialties or 'don't know yet'.

To be a GP you need to get a vocational training certificate. This means training for two years in hospital SHO posts in a GP vocational training scheme or in a series of unlinked, but approved, SHO posts in relevant specialties in a self-constructed or 'DIY' scheme. This latter route often being chosen by those who decide to go into general practice having already started training in another field. See page 74 for more detail.

To become a specialist you need to acquire the entry requirements for specialist registrar training. Each specialty sets its own entry requirements. These usually include at least two years at SHO level, obtaining the relevant experience and passing an examination. If you are sure what you want to do and eager to get on with it then go for a basic training rotation in the specialty of your choice. Try to get one where the supervision and experience are good and SHOs have a record of success in passing their examinations. The grapevine will be fairly accurate or ring up the incumbent SHO. Most will be happy to give you their frank opinion, in confidence.

For those who are not yet certain of their aims, some SHO jobs are useful experience for a variety of careers and give you time to make up your mind before entering a specific career pathway. Accident and Emergency (A&E) posts are a good example. Many doctors choose to do six months in A&E to get some broad experience and self-confidence before applying for a basic specialist rotation. In addition A&E is recognized for most specialties and is excellent preparation for working abroad with a voluntary agency. Some time in general medicine, care of the elderly or general practice is excellent preparation for apparently unrelated careers like surgery or anaesthetics. However if you do spend time like this, be prepared to defend yourself against accusations of indecision or drifting.

SHO training is less tightly controlled than the preregistration year or specialist registrar training, in that there is no time limit on how long you can spend in the grade. However there is an educational management structure overseeing the posts though not the individual doctors. Each Royal College sets standards for SHO training and monitors the quality of the posts by a regular series of hospital visits. There is usually a College tutor for each specialty in each hospital, who is responsible to the College for making sure that the training standards are delivered. The College tutor is an excellent source of advice about courses, study leave, examinations and career pathways in a specialty. For GP vocational trainees there is a GP course organizer who arranges weekly training sessions and offers careers advice. Each hospital will also have a clinical tutor, who usually runs a postgraduate centre where educational events take place, has a say in the running of a library and manages the study leave budget. The clinical tutor is an important figure, who has the ear of the NHS chief executive and the postgraduate dean. He or she is an excellent person to contact for general careers advice, if you are not decided on a specific specialty.

Specialist registrar training

In order to become a consultant you must get your name on the GMC's Specialist Register. Your first step is to look in the *BMJ* or other medical journals for advertised vacancies on training programmes in the specialty or specialties of your choice. The selection procedure is likely to be more rigorous than at SHO level and may be unfamiliar to you. Some appointment panels like to ask the applicants to prepare a short presentation on a topic such as 'How this specialty will develop over the next 10 years' or whatever. Others may request an essay. In one region they video candidates breaking bad news to an actor to assess communication skills. Do whatever is requested of you and if the application form says 'Do not send separate CV', then don't.

If you are lucky enough to be selected, and have right of residence in the UK, you will be given a national training number (NTN). This is your passport to training. Do not lightly relinquish it until you have got your name on the Specialist Register. While you hold your NTN, you are entitled to a series of suitable training placement until your training is complete. If you take time out of programme to do research or to work abroad (always provided you have gained permission from the postgraduate dean) or have a baby, you can do so comfortable in the knowledge that a place in the programme will be found for you on your return. The NTN is specialty specific and provides a passport to training for just one of the 64 recognized specialties in which you can claim a Certificate of Completion of Specialist Training (CCST). It is not easy to move from one specialty to another without competing afresh in you new field. Nor is it that easy to move from one part of the country to another in the same specialty. Although called 'national' the NTNs are issued by regional postgraduate deans who manage their part of the country. While they may give permission for you to transfer your training from one part of the country to another they'll want a pretty good reason for doing so.

Once you have gained a place on a specialty training programme, your training will be managed by a specialty training committee (STC), which is where the postgraduate dean, the Royal College representatives and local consultant trainers come together. The STC will organize an annual review of your progress and generate the appropriate Record of In-Training Assessment (RITA) form. Form A has your personal details and your expected date of getting the CCST. Form B records any subsequent changes to your details. Form C is issued every year if your progress has been satisfactory. Form D indicates that you need targeted training or extra supervision in an area but with no delay to your CCST date. Form E identifies you as requiring repeat experience and delays your CCST date. Form G is issued when your training is expected to be completed within the next three months. On receipt of form G, the STC reviews your records and decides whether to recommend you to the Specialist Training Authority (STA), which in turn hopefully issues you with a CCST, which finally gets you that place on the GMC's Specialist Register, which, in turn, entitles you to be appointed to a consultant position. And you will have earned it!

For further information	Regional Postgraduate Deans and Regional Specialty Advisers
	Regional Postgraduate Advisers in General Practice (i.e. training in general practice)
	The appropriate medical Royal College or Faculty
	The Specialist Training Authority and the General Medical Council

Part-time and flexible training

At any stage from preregistration house officer to specialist registrar level, it is possible to continue your training on a less than full time basis, provided you have well founded reasons for doing so. Over 90% of doctors who choose this pattern of working are women with young families but flexible training is equally available for men with domestic responsibilities. Other common reasons for choosing flexible training include ill-health or disability.

In essence, flexible training is designed to offer the same training as full time training but with reduced weekly hours and therefore it takes longer overall. The flexibility relates to more than the hours, in that the training is tailored to the individual needs of the trainee who may have geographical or other restrictions related to domestic responsibilities or health. Because the training is individually tailored, the funding for the trainee's basic salary usually comes from the postgraduate dean's budget. The trainee is placed in a department that has the capacity to offer the necessary experience and supervision. As an extra pair of hands, you are usually welcome, but you need to make sure that the post delivers the training you need, and that the relevant Royal College has approved the arrangements. The training time is calculated pro-rata, so if you work five sessions a week (the minimum) it will take you twice as long to complete your training.

In most deaneries there is an associate dean who takes special responsibility for flexible training. He or she will offer advice about whether your reason would be considered well founded, put you in touch with someone in your speciality who could give advice, arrange a supernumerary post if appropriate, and make sure that your post is approved by the Royal College. In some cases, especially at SHO level, part-time posts have been established in popular specialities and will be advertised. In other cases, especially in specialities popular with women such as paediatrics, anaesthetics or psychiatry, where flexible training is common, you will be expected to undertake your flexible training by sharing an established post with another flexible trainee. In the surgical specialities flexible training is seen as very strange and you may have to deal with a certain amount of ignorance and a certain amount of suspicion.

If you wish to raise a family and have time with your children and can afford the pro-rata drop in earnings, then some time in flexible training is worth serious thought. Taking it more slowly for a few years need not blight your career. Many of the 'great and the good' trained flexibly at some stage.

Discrimination

This remains widespread throughout medicine. It exists at all levels of the profession and affects a very wide range of people. It is important to distinguish genuine discrimination from the rather more prevalent 'old boy network'.

While it is usually true that the brightest get the best jobs, who you know is often as, if not more, important than what you know. Having said that, dunces are rarely appointed to excellent jobs no matter how well they play rugby.

Discrimination centres on four different levels: application to medical schools, within the college itself, junior jobs, and application for consultant posts. The way different people are discriminated against varies depending on their level within the profession.

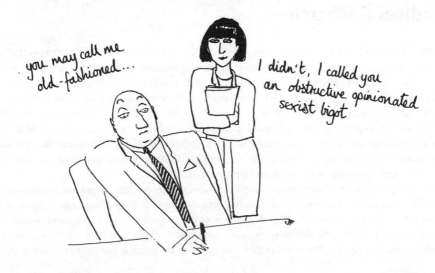

The view of medical college as the preserve of white, middle class, ex-public schoolboys is no longer true. More women than men are now being accepted into medical schools and all colleges are now keen to show that their selection lacks any racial bias. Most medical students are state educated. Whilst those getting into medical school come from the widest posssible background, it remains true that having a medical background can often be an advantage. Medical schools have differing policies on mature students and some, especially in London, are keen to recruit them, but others actively discourage postgraduate applicants. It is worth checking with any individual college before applying.

As a clinical medical student and consequently being lower than a cockroach in the pecking order, it can sometimes feel as if everyone is picking on you. It is worth being sensible about this; students are dependent on firm grades; grades are awarded by consultants and consultants have a wide range of prejudices. Male students with designer stubble and ponytails will often receive lower grades than their less hirsute colleagues. One South London consultant is known to send students off the ward if they are wearing button-down collars as these are apparently too casual. Adapt and survive.

The junior doctor is only as good as his or her last reference; this can lead to 'junior abuse', long hours and excessive workload. This is becoming increasingly less common due to the reforms but talk to the current incumbent of any post before applying. Discriminating dinosaurs still exist and are best avoided—'She's really very good for a girl'.

Specific prejudice exists towards women (see the 'Women in medicine' section below) as well as to 'non-British' doctors. A newly appointed consultant anaesthetist asked his secretary for the CVs of the applicants for the registrar post; she brought through a pile saying 'I've thrown away the ones with funny-sounding surnames'. The anaesthetist found this had been his predecessor's standard practice. I know of at least one colleague who has enjoyed greater success with job applications since having his name anglicized by deed poll.

It is on applying for a consultant post that many have hit their heads on the 'glass ceiling'. This exists for women (especially in surgery) and gay men. Some are held back by reputations of which they may be entirely unaware.

Having said all this, the determined and the good will always get to the top eventually. The brilliant get there even more quickly, regardless of colour, gender or sexuality.

Medical Research

A career in medicine attracts the most gifted students. *Tomorrow's Doctors* (GMC 1993) states that learning should be promoted 'through curiosity, the exploration of knowledge, and the critical evaluation of evidence'. It naturally follows, despite the demands of the undergraduate curriculum, that many will question the assertions that are made by their teachers (all too often presented as 'fact') and wish to examine the quality of the evidence which has led to those assertions. The intellectual challenges posed by our limited understanding of the factors that are essential for the maintenance and improvement of human health, together with humanitarian motives, will lead many medical graduates to consider a career in research so that they may make a direct contribution to improving the prevention, diagnosis and treatment of disease.

A majority of those in training grades who are following a service career track are encouraged to gain some experience of research. This is an important element in the postgraduate training of all doctors and is essential for instilling the disciplines which are necessary for a lifetime of continuing self-education. It enables the doctor to evaluate published material, facilitates the transfer of new developments to proven value into practice and qualifies the practitioner to participate in audit activities and to collaborate in research activities. All these will contribute directly to the development of the service (e.g. trials or epidemiological studies). The nature of the necessary research training for those who plan to follow a service career is specified by the relevant Royal Colleges and their specialist advisory committees.

A smaller proportion of medical graduates will have ambitions to develop a major career in medical research. A wide range of opportunities is open to this group, ranging from the molecular sciences to research on individual patients and populations. Many will take the first steps towards a research career during their undergraduate years by taking an intercalated BSc (or enrolling in an MB/PhD programme) or undertaking a significant research project.

Training and career development

Research training during the postgraduate period requires a substantial commitment on the part of the trainee. It must be regarded as a full-time activity requiring at least two years or, more normally, three years in order to acquire the necessary skills and experience that are the necessary first steps towards establishing a career as an independent investigator. Many will also require an additional period when holding a career development award, to develop their research interests and their clinical or public health career further before being in a position to acquire a senior post. It is generally possible to make arrangements which will enable the trainee to acquire the necessary clinical or pubic health experience to meet the requirement of the Royal Colleges in order to acquire the CCST and gain entry to the specialist register at the same time—although the process may take one or two years longer than the minimum time for acquisition of the CCST envisaged by the new specialist registrar training arrangements. It is essential that trainees discuss these with their postgraduate dean, Royal College and research funding body at the outset. Remuneration for those undertaking research training fellowships and career development awards equate with those paid to trainees following a service career track.

Career posts and opportunities

Medical research takes place in many different places—universities, hospitals, general practice, research institutes and industry. Opportunities at senior levels are available in all these environments. The majority are likely to develop their careers within a university setting (as senior lecturer, reader or professor) or within research institutes and the majority of these offer similar career opportunities and salaries—and often senior researchers are awarded academic status since the majority of these are associated with universities. Appropriate honorary clinical status (i.e. consultant) is almost invariably awarded to all at this level of seniority.

Financial rewards

Salary scales are equivalent to those available with the NHS (for clinical academic staff) and the university system (for those in research institutes or units). Those with honorary consultant contracts are also eligible for NHS distinction awards.

Advice

It is essential that all those thinking of pursuing a research career should obtain appropriate advice. This should cover issues such as areas for research, the development of suitable projects for research training, training opportunities, the identification of an appropriate training environment and the interaction of research and clinical training requirements. It should be remembered that advice can be good or bad and it is generally desirable to take advice from a number of sources. It is essential that advice should be taken from the postgraduate dean and the appropriate Royal College for all those planning a clinical research career and from the major research funding body.

Funding

The two largest sources of funding for medical research in Britain, and for research training and career development awards, are the Medical Research Council and the Wellcome Trust. However, funds are also available from many other sources, including other research charities and a number of local and private funds. Training and career development awards have to be won in competition from the research funding bodies.

Conclusion

Medical research is always interesting, intellectually challenging and highly competitive. The rewards are considerable and include the opportunity to make significant contributions to the development of clinical and public health practice, to meet and work as a member or leader of a team with intellectually able and stimulating people (frequently from other disciplines) and to gain membership of the informal international club which draws research scientists with common interests from all parts of the world.

For further information	**Heads of Programmes, Career and Clinical Initiatives** Wellcome Trust 183 Euston Road London NW1 4SP Tel: 020 7611 8888 Fax: 020 7611 8545 Website: www.wellcome.ac.uk
	Training Awards Group Medical Research Council 20 Park Crescent London W1N 4AL
	General Secretary Association of Medical Research Charities 29–35 Farringdon Road London EC1M 3JB Tel: 020 7404 6454 Fax: 020 7404 6448 Website: www.amrc.org.uk

Women in medicine

Two years ago, when writing for the first edition, I questioned whether a special section for women was still relevant. Although we have progressed a lot since I trained, I now realize that we have merely pushed the glass ceiling higher. Only recently, as a fairly senior consultant, has my head pushed up against it again—but it feels and looks the same as the one I pushed against as a student and junior doctor. We have congratulated ourselves in recent years that the number of female consultants has increased. Sadly, recent figures published by the Women in Surgical Training Scheme (WIST) show that women's percentage representation in some surgical specialties has actually decreased, the increase in numbers being merely a reflection of moves towards consultant expansion. For a while we had a female President of a Royal College in Fiona Caldicott at the Royal College of Psychiatrists, but even this did not allow full discussion of women's issues at the highest level. Dame Fiona speaks of 'women's issues' at College Presidents' meetings being deferred to later meetings—after she had stepped down, and where no senior woman would be present.

It is now accepted that women can become consultants, but to progress beyond that is not so accepted. Committee work often demands evenings devoted to not very exciting meetings and late returns home. Until more women are represented on committees the meetings will not change, nor will attitudes. If we are to change the profession for the better, the importance of committees and College business must be recognized and a culture of 'she's off skiving at another meeting' must be banished forever.

So is this relevant to you as medical students? The message for today is that there are probably sufficient rules and regulations to ensure fair play at more junior levels. Those of us who fought to establish those rights are now in their forties and fifties, and we continue to push for equality for all, right up to the top of the profession, but there are quite a few battles left to fight.

I am still concerned that female medical students seek me out when they are on elective placements in my hospital. They want to meet me and still tell tales of how they are being put off a

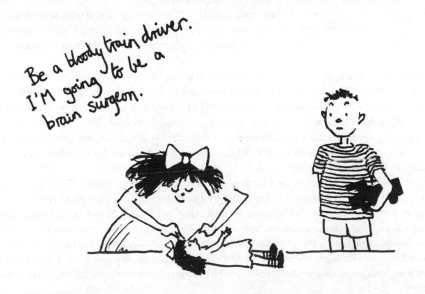

surgical career by their advisers in medical school. In October 1998, at a meeting of women doctors in Oxford, there was general acknowledgement that these attitudes are still prevalent. Today's students are not being advised by elderly surgical dinosaurs, but by dynamic young consultants who allow themselves to express the prejudices that should have been buried along with the older generation who have now passed on. Medical schools are now admitting at least 50% female students, on the basis that they have the same freedom of career choice on qualifying as their male counterparts, and in theory at least there is no job which is not open to women. The most quoted objections to training and employment are obviously related to the issues of child-bearing but not all women want to have children and for those who do not it is extremely frustrating to see all issues relating to equality of opportunity expressed in terms of maternity leave and flexible training. It is personally insulting not to be believed when one has made such a decision, or to feel obliged to explain if one physically cannot have children for whatever reason. We still have to find ways to head off such intrusive enquiries into our private lives without giving offence. I do not believe one method will apply to all, but more formalized personnel rules, which state quite clearly what information can be asked of potential job applicants, will help enormously. If one wishes to make a career in general practice, many vocational training schemes and part-time posts exist. Many practices regard it as desirable to have at least one female partner if not more. With a moderate amount of flexibility and co-operation with one's partners, good job satisfaction can generally be obtained.

I believe that most job satisfaction will come from doing whatever it is that one most enjoys. After each clinical attachment, as a medical student, perhaps one should ask 'Did I enjoy that?' and 'Was I reasonably good at that?' It is easy at the end of a popular attachment to get sidetracked or to want to do every specialty as one gets to grips with it. However, if you are still attracted to a particular subject after a variety of clinical firms, then that is something that will be really enjoyable in the long term. Consider doing an elective in a related department in another hospital or another country and find out as much as you can about your clinical interest. Never allow yourself to be put off by comments such as 'That's no good for women' or 'That's a far too macho specialty for you'.

In the past some women have made the mistake of trying to be like men when they choose 'macho' specialties. There is no specialty which requires stereotypically male behaviour in isolation. Today's patients have a high level of communication with their hospital specialist and the use of one's own communication skills, in a way which is appropriate to one's gender, should never be underestimated. It is not necessary to wear trousers or a pinstriped suit to function as a good consultant.

A male and female surgeon may deal with the issue of giving bad news in a totally different way. In some cultures it would be inappropriate for a male doctor to shed a tear with a patient; in the same culture a female doctor who cries with a patient may be considered human and sympathetic and does help the patient to cope. Patients are becoming more sophisticated all the time and are very good at picking up insincerity and pomposity. It is important to be oneself and openly admit that one does not know all the answers. A patient may perceive that you are being honest, and this is important in all good communication.

Because women tend to live longer than men, over 50% of patients are female. There is also still a tendency for children to be brought to the doctor by a mother or other female relative, while child-bearing and its sequelae may lead to more frequent visits over a number of years. Some female patients will prefer to see a male doctor, but many will be glad to talk to another woman. Women doctors should capitalize on this to make a patient more at ease—yet again, just be yourself. If you are considering combining medicine and having a family, it is generally much easier than it might seem at first. Teaching, a traditionally good profession for women, has done little to keep women in the workplace before their own children reach school age. A five year break is too long for any serious career woman, especially where fine manual skills and up-to-date knowledge are required. The medical profession has recognized the need to allow women (and men) who wish to work part-time to keep their skills current by 'flexible training' or the older 'women's retainer' schemes. If you have a skill, it is important not to lose it and practising that skill for a very few hours a week can prevent it being lost. Flexible training means that a trainee must work at least half-time (at any grade) with pro-rata on-call commitments. The time to get the experience may thus be twice as long as in a full-time post.

The way to investigate this scheme is to get an information pack from the relevant Royal College and to contract the postgraduate dean's office to find out about training approval, funding and availability in any geographical region. Flexible training posts may take longer to organize than part-time posts so plan ahead. A new difficulty has occurred in the specialist training scheme. Removal of supernumerary status from some part-time and flexible training posts has, once again, put women who are contemplating a family at a disadvantage. One hopes that this retrograde step is only temporary but further work needs to be done to re-establish the right to train at an appropriate rate to one's personal circumstances. In surgery, long regarded as the last bastion of male chauvinism, the Royal College of Surgeons of England has established WIST to banish this myth and has organized a national network and mutual support groups. Every region has at least one representative who is a consultant surgeon committed to helping women train in surgery. Often these WIST representatives liaise with mentors in other specialties and help women trainees in other fields, or refer them on to other approachable consultants who have experience in dealing with the problems of a particular non-surgical specialty. The Medical Women's Federation also exists to help women in medicine in all disciplines and at all career stages by providing mutual support and sensible careers advice.

After training you may wish to work part-time. It is not unusual to seek and obtain a part-time post in the NHS at consultant level and many male consultants choose to work part-time for the NHS and spend time in private practice. Some women may not wish to study for higher qualifications or wish to progress to consultant responsibility and sub-consultant grades such as staff grade and associate specialist posts may provide the answer, but the job satisfaction *per se* or the status of such posts may be lower than that of the career posts.

Issues surrounding recognition of these sub-consultant grades are currently very much in the national/political agenda. Part-time training schemes and any 'unusual training route' were originally seen as back-door routes to higher training posts. It is as important to be honest with yourself as it is with your patients. Try not to use a part-time post purely to buy time before taking an examination. These schemes are set up to ensure equality and must not be seen as a way to bypass reasonable career obstacles that are there in order to maintain high professional standards. It is important as ever to be as good as the male candidate.

For further information	**Women in Surgical Training** The Royal College of Surgeons of England 35–43 Lincoln's Inn Fields London WC2A 3PN Tel: 020 7869 6212 Fax: 020 7831 9438 Website: www.rcseng.ac.uk/training/wist

Medical Women's Federation
Tavistock House North
Tavistock Square
London WC1H 9HX
Tel: 020 7387 7765
Website: www.m-w-f.demon.co.uk

CHAPTER 2

Surgery

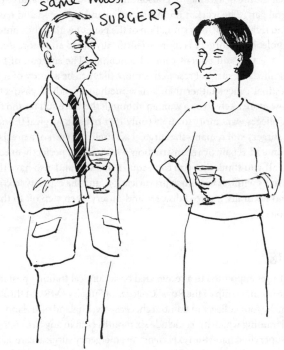

Come come, Margaret. You are surely not implying that if women are better at the fiddly bits on an assembly line, that the same must be true for SURGERY?

Overview

There is a stereotyped image of a surgeon which seems to originate from old Ealing comedies and the *Doctor in the House* series of books by Richard Gordon. The bluff James Robertson Justice type is met at the hospital front door by his obsequious team of junior staff who present him with a fresh red carnation for his buttonhole before the ward round. In the hospital he is king and conqueror, is answerable to no one and is rude to everyone, in particular the patients. Yet he is tolerated and, in some circles, admired because he is a quick, safe, and excellent technician and is always available at any hour for any patient in trouble.

Even in contemporary TV soap operas the macho image of the surgical consultant remains. He is a man (of course), knife-happy, still offensively rude and exploits a sort of *droit de seigneur* by bonking nurses and any other willing hospital handmaidens during nights on-call. Yet his empire has now contracted. The surgeon may still think he can rule the roost in the operating theatre but the rules are different and the patronizing pat on the bottom of a theatre nurse will now lead to a disciplinary action.

The facts are that the life of a trainee or consultant is as a member of a large team where each plays an essential integral part. The work is more structured and regulated and has to take into account the sensitivities and rights to self-determination of the patient within the context of the provision of healthcare as a whole. Also, surgery is more scientifically based and more dependent on audit and measurement of objective and patient-centred outcomes. The surgeon of today is much more a physician with a knife, and surgical research is more likely to be a study of matrix metalloproteinases in gastrointestinal cancer rather than a new method of radical gastrectomy for cancer. The surgeon is also now more likely to be a woman although there are still far too few women in surgery and the surgical Colleges want more to apply (only 15% of basic surgical trainees are women).

The essence of surgery still remains the surgical act itself; the craft of a precise anatomical surgical dissection, excision and repair or reconstruction which, when perfectly executed, always brings a tingle to the spine. If you think that you can acquire this skill and also have the ability to make the best possible decisions without too much prevarication, and the capacity to cope with the occasional self-induced and naturally induced disaster and misery, then step on to the bottom rung of the ladder of your choice.

Early training

The first move is to get appointed to a recognized basic surgical training post before applying to take the diploma of the Membership of the Royal Colleges of Surgery (MRCS) through the relevant training board of *one* of the four colleges in Edinburgh, Glasgow, England or Ireland. There then follow two years of approved training which must include six months each in any two Category I posts, which are jobs that involve supervised hands-on experience in emergency surgical care such as a general surgical post with emergency work, trauma and orthopaedics or accident and emergency medicine. The next 12 months can be spent in approved jobs of your choice which may be within the Category I bracket or in Category II such as neurosurgery, ENT or urology, but make sure that you do not spend more than six months in any one. You will be observed and supervised during these years and must earn a satisfactory assessment at the end of each term including scrutiny of your logbook. Bear in mind that although a demonstrator's post in anatomy is time well spent it does not count towards clinical training although there may be exceptions which are tied up with an accident and emergency job.

Surgery: career pathway

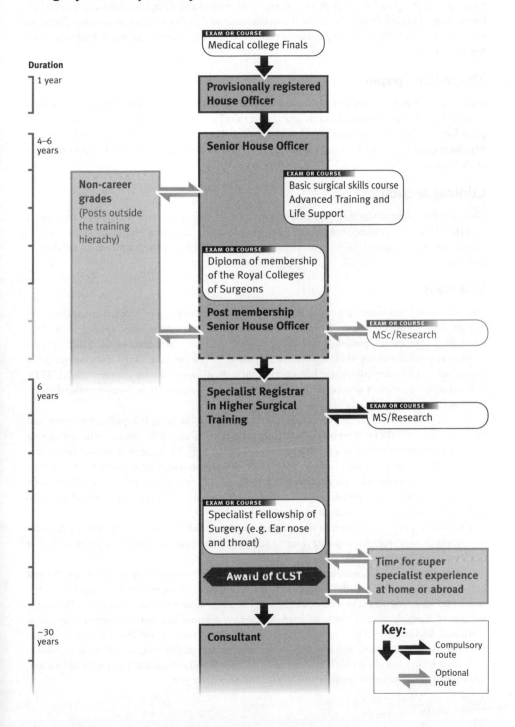

Duration

1 year

4–6 years

6 years

~30 years

EXAM OR COURSE
Medical college Finals

Provisionally registered House Officer

Senior House Officer

EXAM OR COURSE
Basic surgical skills course
Advanced Training and Life Support

Non-career grades
(Posts outside the training hierachy)

EXAM OR COURSE
Diploma of membership of the Royal Colleges of Surgeons

Post membership Senior House Officer

EXAM OR COURSE
MSc/Research

Specialist Registrar in Higher Surgical Training

EXAM OR COURSE
MS/Research

EXAM OR COURSE
Specialist Fellowship of Surgery (e.g. Ear nose and throat)

Award of CCST

Time for super specialist experience at home or abroad

Consultant

Key:
Compulsory route
Optional route

The first postgraduate surgical examination of MRCS assesses fundamental surgical skills and training. The integrated syllabus of basic science and clinical knowledge has been approved by all four colleges but varies a little in format (for details refer to the relevant College website). There are three parts of the MRCS exam which can be taken separately at intervals throughout training or all together at the end:

The written paper

There are two papers the first of which covers the core modules and the second the system modules. At least a third of all questions in both papers cover the basic sciences of anatomy, physiology and pathology. Each paper contains 90 minutes of true/false question and 30 minutes of extended matching questions which is thought to be a better test of knowledge than the old five-part multiple choice questions.

Clinical section

The exam lasts about an hour and is based on a mixture of 'short cases' seen in five bays covering (i) superficial lesions, (ii) musculoskeletal and neurosurgery, (iii) circulation and lymphatic, (iv) trunk and (v) communication skills. This part of the exam is usually taken in the last six months of clinical training.

The vivas

You must have completed 22 months in approved posts before the *viva voce* section of three 20-minute oral exams covering applied surgical anatomy and operative surgery, applied physiology and critical care, clinical pathology and the principles of surgery. You can take the written papers as often as you like but the whole exam must be passed within two years of the first attempt of the clinical section. The English College of Surgery launched a distance learning course in 1996 (STEP–MRCS) which provides a structured learning programme alongside clinical duties without interrupting the flow of training.

After MRCS you are in a position to apply for higher surgical training as a specialist registrar and then enrolling with the joint committee of higher surgical training. All the specialties have a six year training programme including a flexible year which can be used for research or further experience in a related surgical area which could involve an overseas secondment. After four years you can sit the specialty fellowship exam, for example FRCS Orthopaedics or FRCS Neurosurgery, which allows you to be included on the specialist registrar of the GMC with a CCST to prove it. Then all you have to do is be appointed to a consultant post!

To avoid too much repetition in the surgical sections which follow, only the specific requirements within each specialist registrar training scheme will be discussed. Here is a broad outline of the training ladder from house officer to consultant.

All this may be a fairly seamless and well organized system but two bottlenecks remain: the first between acquisition of the MRCS diploma and appointment to a specialist programme and the second for an appointment to a consultant post. The surgical establishment recognizes the disadvantage of hanging around too long after completing training and have convened a specialist workforce advisory group seeking early placement. But one has to accept that high standards are maintained not only by a rigorous and effectively monitored training programme but also by competitive elements. It is always likely that the early bottleneck will remain but if you want to be a surgeon you are likely to be competitive so don't let anything deter you.

For further information

Royal College of Surgeons of England
35/43 Lincoln's Inn Fields
London WC2A 3PN
Tel: 020 7405 3474
Fax: 020 7831 9438
Website: www.rcseng.ac.uk

Royal College of Physicians and Surgeons of Glasgow
232–242 St Vincent Street
Glasgow G2 5RJ
Tel: 0141 221 6072
Fax: 0141 221 1804
Website: www.rcpsglasg.ac.uk

Royal College of Surgeons of Ireland
St Stephen's Green
Dublin 2
Tel: 00 353 1 402 2100
Website: www.rcsi.ie/

Royal College of Surgeons of Edinburgh
Nicolson Street
Edinburgh EH8 9DW
Tel: 0131 527 1600
Fax: 0131 557 6406
Website: www.rcsed.ac.uk

Breast surgery/surgical oncology

Sixty per cent of those people who are cured of the common solid cancers (lung, breast, bowel, etc.) are cured by surgery alone. Of the other 40%, a small number are cured by radiotherapy or chemotherapy (alone or in combination) and the vast majority by the combination of one or both of these modalities with surgery. Surgical oncology in the UK is not yet recognized as a distinct entity but it is expected that more surgeons will devote the whole of their practice to the management of patients with cancer and cancer-related illnesses.

The role of the surgical oncologist has been best defined, in the UK, by the development of breast surgery. Following the implementation of the Calman–Hyne proposals on the delivery of cancer care, most general hospitals in the UK have developed integrated breast units to manage women with a wide range of breast disorders (only one in 15 women who fear that they might have breast cancer, actually have the disease). In most centres every effort is made to achieve a diagnosis on the day of attendance in collaboration with colleagues in radiology and cytopathology. For those women who are found to have breast cancer, their further management would be jointly between the surgeon, the radiotherapist and the medical oncologist. Cancer patients need much more time than most other patients, helped as necessary by nurse counsellors.

Pure breast surgery at present only exists in a small number of major university centres. Most breast surgeons have a secondary interest and while many jobs are advertised for breast and endocrine surgery, the majority have a secondary interest in surgical gastroenterology.

After successfully completing the basic surgical training, the six-year specialist training rotation begins. While year 4 of this programme is usually reserved for a period of research, competition is such that many successful candidates for specialist registrar appointments already have undertaken a Doctorate of Medicine (MD) thesis. The first three years of this rotation would be in the generality of surgery, while the last two years (during which time the candidate will sit the intercollegiate FRCS examination) would be undertaken in a specialist breast unit. Since a large proportion of breast cancer patients have a family history of breast cancer, some training in the science of genetics and molecular biology is needed to keep up-to-date with current management strategies. Presently, an appointment as a consultant breast surgeon will usually involve an on-call commitment on the general surgical rota and the successful candidate would be expected to demonstrate the ability to manage the acute abdomen and trauma.

Other areas where oncological surgery predominate include thoracic surgery (lung and oesophagus), upper gastrointestinal surgery (oesophagus, stomach, pancreas and liver), colorectal surgery and some parts of orthopaedic and plastic and reconstructive surgery. If the consultant surgeon elects to undertake a large volume of cancer surgery in any of these disciplines, he/she must structure their job plan accordingly. Although there are depressions and huge disappointments when cancer is incurable, there can be immense rewards from both successful curative operations and successful palliative surgery to restore the quality of a patient's life. Here liaison with the palliative medical service is invaluable.

Myth	They only do radical mastectomies.
Reality	An extremely demanding job with a difficult and wide variety of surgery.
Personality	More compassion than most.
Best aspects	Thanks to the National Screening Programme, breast cancer is being detected earlier. Possibility for cure and even eradication of the disease.
Worst aspects	High volume of outpatient work. Tremendous emotional commitment to both patients and relatives.
Requirements	FRCS and MS/MD

Hours

Junior   Consultant

Numbers   350 in total (50 per year)   10% are women and increasing

Competitiveness

Stress

On-calls

Junior   Consultant

Salary   £60 000   £75 000   £200 000

For further information
British Association of Surgical Oncology
Royal College of Surgeons of England
35–43 Lincoln's Inn Fields
London WC2A 3PN
Tel: 020 7405 5612
Fax: 020 7404 6574
Website: www.baso.org

Cardiothoracic surgery

Cardiac surgery is expanding. The recent National Service framework for coronary heart disease aims to approximately double the number of coronary bypass operations performed annually over the next ten years to bring us into line with other developed health economies. As part of this initiative the number of training posts has been significantly increased but the specialty is very competitive and it is necessary to make yourself very marketable to secure an NTN. Cardiothoracic surgical training now takes six years with an optional year for research. Whilst this is an appropriate length of time to train in this specialty, you are unlikely to have an easy passage from SHO to NTN without spending some time in the specialty beforehand. Once the MRCS or equivalent is passed there are several options:

- spending more time as a senior SHO whilst applying for NTN posts;
- going into a research post and doing some clinical work;
- obtaining a locum post (for training or service (LATS or LAS)) while waiting for NTN posts.

Once you have gained an NTN the hard work really begins. Cardiothoracic surgery has been fighting a rearguard action to keep longer working hours. This is not because we want the trainees to work any longer than other specialties but because a great deal of cardiothoracic surgery is based on clinical experience and if you are not around then you will not get the experience.

There are now rigorous annual assessments called Records of In-Training Assessment (RITA) which have to be passed before progression to the next year is allowed. Time off the rotation is permitted for research and overseas experience (subject to approval from the Specialty Advisory Committee (SAC)) in cardiothoracic surgery. After year 4 you are permitted to sit the intercollegiate specialty exam (Part III) which is an exam with a pass rate of about 50% for each sitting. On entering year 6 you should know when your CCST date is due and once this is approved you can begin to apply for consultant posts.

Most rotations have a specific slot for thoracic surgery which includes pulmonary, oesophageal surgery and chest wall surgery. Cardiac surgical training generally revolves around adult surgery with subspecialist training in paediatric cardiac surgery and cardiopulmonary transplantation. The majority choose to pursue a consultant post in cardiac or cardiothoracic surgery whilst a few choose a career in thoracic surgery. Although thoracic surgery may not appear as glamorous as cardiac surgery, it is certainly much more varied and even more challenging than routine adult cardiac surgery.

Cardiac surgeons have been the first group of clinicians to have their surgical results scrutinized. This aspect of the job adds considerably to the stress of the job and is likely to get worse as the patient population changes. One consequence of such forensic scrutiny is that the practice of cardiothoracic surgery has become increasingly consultant-based. A second is greater consultant supervision of training. In addition, as a result of technological innovation, the clinical face of cardiac surgery will change over the next few years with more focus on minimally invasive procedures, including robotics, and surgery adapted to the treatment of heart failure.

Cardiothoracic surgery may be demanding and highly competitive but it is technically fascinating and, clinically, very rewarding.

Myth	'Balls of steel' surgeons who love the sight of blood.
Reality	An expanding specialty with a good career structure. Rewarding surgery in terms of technique and patient satisfaction. Consultant-led specialty with the emphasis on training juniors.
Personality	Very varied, occasional megalomaniacs.
Best aspects	The surgery, intensive therapy unit experience and grateful patients.
Worst aspects	Terror—patients can deteriorate very quickly.
Requirements	FRCS

Hours

Junior   Consultant

Numbers   220 (10 per year)   3% are women

Competitiveness

Stress

On-calls

Junior   **Consultant:** can be variable but consultant-requiring emergencies are common

Salary   £50 000   £130 000   £500 000

For further information   **Society of Cardiothoracic Surgeons of Great Britain and Ireland**
Royal College of Surgeons of England
35–43 Lincoln's Inn Fields
London WC2A 3PN
Tel: 020 7405 3474
Fax: 020 7831 9438
Website: www.scts.org

Coloproctology and upper gastrointestinal surgery (including hepatobiliary surgery)

Many general surgeons specialize in a specific area such as the gastrointestinal (GI) tract. Sub-specialization often goes further, concentrating on the upper GI tract (oesophagus, stomach, hepatobiliary and pancreas) or coloproctology (colon, rectum and anus). General surgery and an on-call emergency commitment form part of the workload.

After the MRCS exam comes the bottleneck into a regional programme of specialist registrar training involving a minimum of five years in clinical posts, plus a flexible year for research or further specialist experience. Increasingly specialist registrars are spending the first two years in general surgical training mainly in district general hospitals. By this time a decision will have been made about subspecialization, and at least one of the final years should be spent in a specialist unit, either coloproctology, upper GI tract and/or hepatobiliary. Some surgeons hope to superspecialize and are encouraged to spend a further year in another unit either in this country or overseas. On the other hand, a surgeon may wish to remain more general, developing expertise in both upper and lower GI tract surgery, especially if the ultimate goal is to be a consultant surgeon in a district general hospital rather than a teaching hospital.

If there are problems 'getting a number' as an specialist registrar due to the bottleneck, the research year can be spent either in the UK or overseas at this time. The aim is to produce a thesis leading to an MD or an MSc, which can be a big advantage when applying for specialist registrar training or a consultant post in such a competitive field but is not mandatory.

The qualities needed to be an upper GI tract or colorectal surgeon include resilience, organizational ability and potential to cope with stress. It is vital that a surgeon is a team player because much of the day-to-day work is shared with colleagues in related disciplines. Apart from manual precision and dexterity, physical and mental fitness is essential because intense concentration is required over several hours.

A surgeon does not necessarily have to be an academic genius, although some are. The latter tend to pursue a career in academic surgery but most choose a more practical career in the NHS, spending part of their time in private practice, although clinical research can still be carried out and is actively encouraged. A special effort is needed to maintain outside interests, although this is difficult sometimes due to the demands of the profession.

A typical week for a consultant surgeon will be one specialist and one general outpatient clinic, three or four operating lists (one of which might be devoted to daycare surgery), an upper GI endoscopy or colonoscopy session and ward rounds. An emergency on-take day rotates with colleagues about once a week, with weekend cover every six to eight weeks. Teaching trainees and undergraduates, administration and private practice (usually one clinic and one operating session, often 'out of hours') also need to be fitted in. Audit of operative results is now an essential part of the job with so much current emphasis on quality and performance (clinical governance).

Myth	James Robertson Justice types spending all their time on the golf course or in private practice, or both.
Reality	Very busy, but very satisfying. The majority of young trainees will progress to consultant status ensuring job security. There is a major trend towards subspecialization in upper GI surgery/hepatobiliary or coloproctology.
Personality	Usually extrovert, good communicators, plenty of stamina, tenacious, manually dextrous.
Best aspects	Technical and intellectual demands of operating and decision-making with early evidence of results. Very practical specialty. Infinitely variable with never a moment of boredom. Excellent patient contact. High job satisfaction. Multidisciplinary team working. Good opportunity for private practice.
Worst aspects	Heavy workload tends to disrupt family and social life. Need an understanding spouse with the patience of Job. Stress caused by insufficient time to do everything. Increasing expectations of patients and Government with insufficient resources to satisfy.
Requirements	FRCS. A high degree (MS, MD, PhD or MSc) a major advantage.

Hours

Junior: restricted by law, many would prefer more experience at this level. This is especially true of surgery.

Consultant: Private practice often 'out of hours'.

Numbers 667 posts 11% women

Competitiveness

Stress

On-calls

Junior

Consultant

Salary

£min £av £max

£50 000 £100 000 £300 000

For further information	**Association of Coloproctology** 35–43 Lincoln's Inn Fields London WC2A 3PN Tel: 020 7973 0307 Fax: 020 7430 9235 Website: www.acpgbi.org.uk	**Association of Upper Gastrointestinal Surgeons of Great Britain and Ireland** 35–43 Lincoln's Inn Fields London WC2A 3PN Tel: 020 7973 0305 Fax: 020 7430 9235

Ear, nose and throat surgery (otorhinolaryngology)

This is a specialty that has undergone a meteoric rise in status and scope. The range of operations is immense and extends from delicate microsurgery inside the ear through to major resections of head and neck cancers, hence the new name otorhinolaryngology.

Ear, nose and throat (ENT) surgery represents over 20% of the GP's workload with a correspondingly great variety of specialist referrals. Within ENT it is possible to develop special interests. Examples include head and neck cancer, cosmetic surgery, voice disorders, endoscopic nasal surgery, sleep disorders and skull base surgery.

The surgery is intimately linked with the advances in sensory physiology and new technology. For instance, knowledge of the inner ear physiology has led to cochlear implantation, insertion of an electrode allowing totally deaf people to hear. ENT surgeons were the first to use the operating microscope in 1921 and now over 50% of ENT operations are done with a microscope or fibre-optic telescope. The use of microscopic and endoscopic techniques, combined with high-resolution radiology and lasers, allows access to the most remote nooks and crannies in the head. The otorhinolaryngologist needs good co-ordination and fine manipulative skills, together with a thorough knowledge of head and neck anatomy, and in this specialty the surgeon is his own physician.

Exposure to ENT in medical school is short. Therefore, before definitely deciding on a career in ENT an SHO job in the specialty is helpful. After that careful career planning is essential. Experience in general surgery (one year) and/or plastic surgery (six months) and/or neurosurgery (six months) is desirable.

After the basic MRCS exam the specialist registrar will spend six years rotating between posts on a regional training programme. The training and experience are recorded and assessed in a logbook and are graded from simpler procedures in the first year to more complex in the final year, taking into account rhinology, otology, surgery of the mouth pharynx and oesophagus, laryngology, endoscopy, head and neck oncology and surgery of salivary glands and structures of the neck. Even if a trainee does not want to take up the option of a research year it is still expected that, for training purposes, they should carry out at least three audit projects under supervision where the outcomes of patient management are assessed, and at least one research project which must be presented to a regional or national professional meeting and accepted for publication.

Myth	It's all snot and wax!
Reality	The most diverse range of surgery available. Hard work, 8 a.m. to 6 p.m.
Personality	Varies from the obsessional (otologist) to the complete hero (head and neck surgeon)
Best aspects	Varied and challenging. Happy, sane patients of all ages. Well-organized training with access to the best surgical toys. A life outside the operating theatre is possible. Well rewarded.
Worst aspects	Huge demand for otolaryngology services with departments generally understaffed. Most competitive specialty in the USA with Britain not far behind.
Requirements	FRCS(Otolaryngology)

Hours

Junior ⏰⏰⏰ Consultant ⏰⏰⏰

Numbers 475 posts   10–15% women

Competitiveness 🗡🗡🗡🗡🗡

Stress ☹☹

On-calls

Junior 📟📟 Consultant 📟📟

Salary

£60 000   £120 000   £500 000

For further information	**British Association of Otolaryngologists** Royal College of Surgeons of England 35–43 Lincoln's Inn Fields London WC2A 3PN Tel: 020 7404 8373 Fax: 020 7404 4200 Website: www.orl-baohns.org

Head and neck surgery

This fascinating branch of surgery is not yet recognized as a stand-alone specialty in the UK. Consequently, most head and neck surgeons commence their career in ENT surgery and then subspecialize during their time in the registrar grade. A minority come into head and neck surgery via plastic or maxillofacial surgery.

Head and neck tumours are comparatively rare thus only teaching centres and larger district general hospitals can realistically support a head and neck service. The optimum requirements for such a service are a head and neck surgeon, a plastic/reconstructive surgeon, a maxillofacial surgeon, a neurosurgeon and a radiotherapist. A medical oncologist is also essential as are a Macmillan nurse, speech therapist and dietitian. Ideally, all should have fixed sessional commitments at the service site.

A thorough knowledge of the relevant anatomy and physiology of the head and neck region is essential. A good 'pair of hands', an ability to manage the ill patient and an understanding of the principles of radiotherapy and chemotherapy are also necessary.

Despite many surgical advances over the last two decades, the five-year survival rate for patients with head and neck malignancies has not altered significantly. Indeed, many patients are obviously beyond the realm of surgical cure at the time of presentation. Therefore, it is also an advantage if the surgeon has the insight and background to care for the terminally ill patient.

Having decided on a career in head and neck surgery, six-month periods in the relevant specialties of ENT, plastic surgery and neurosurgery within the basic surgical training years will prove invaluable, as will a period in a general surgical post that offers good practical experience. The trainee may, therefore, wish to create his or her own training scheme at this level, or a pre-existing scheme can be adapted to fit the individual's requirements.

The most appropriate higher surgical training scheme is in ENT surgery. However, no scheme will provide comprehensive training in head and neck surgery; the deficit must therefore be made by spending a year or more in an established head and neck unit which can be arranged during or after the higher surgical training period. There are many excellent units abroad which regularly take Fellows from the UK. Whilst it is advantageous to develop a research interest within the specialty, clinical experience is more important in the end.

Having achieved specialist accreditation and passed the third, 'exit' examination in ENT, or possibly plastic surgery, the hunt then begins for a consultant job either with an established head and neck surgery interest or one with potential. Take your time and be very selective.

Myth	Knife-happy, 'the bigger the tumour the better' surgeons.
Reality	A small specialty which relies on co-operation with various allied disciplines. Has reached the end of the line with regard to pure surgical development.
Personality	Level-headed, thoughtful and with an ability to say no.
Best aspects	Varied spectrum of diseases, not all malignant. Fascinating anatomy. Incorporates the expertise of many disciplines. Molecular biology aspect expanding rapidly.
Worst aspects	Many patients present with advanced disease, so the overall survival rate is poor, which can be very depressing. Still awaiting proper recognition as a specialty of its own.
Requirements	FRCS

Hours

🕐 🕐 🕐 🕐 🕐   🕐 🕐 🕐 🕐 🕐

Junior   Consultant

Numbers	80 consultants 3 per year currently very few are women

Competitiveness

🗡 🗡 🗡 🗡 🗡

Stress

☹ ☹ ☹ ☹ ☹

On-calls

📟 📟 📟 📟 📟   📟 📟 📟 📟 📟

Junior   Consultant

Salary

£min   £av   £max

£50 000   £80 000   £150 000

For further information

British Association of Otolaryngologists
Royal College of Surgeons of England
35–43 Lincoln's Inn Fields
London WC2A 3PN
Tel: 020 7405 8373
Fax: 020 7404 4200
Website: www.orl-baohns.org

Maxillofacial surgery

This branch of surgery has changed out of all recognition following its conception over 40 years ago, arising from the management of facial injuries by dental practitioners within the hospital services. The initial stimulus from this work came from the severe facial injuries caused by the two World Wars. It soon became apparent that the skills of these specialists could be used to treat the diverse number of conditions within the head and neck area and the discipline of maxillofacial surgery was founded and has been one of the forerunners of the current concept of anatomically based surgery.

The training is long and arduous as the maxillofacial surgeon must achieve both dental and medical qualifications. Most surgeons entering this discipline are dental graduates. As from the year 2003 the training pathway to a consultant in maxillofacial surgery will be redefined. After a Bachelor's degree in dental surgery or an equivalent dental degree, two years' general professional training will be required at the house officer (HO) or SHO level in a maxillofacial surgery department, with the passing of the examination to become a member of the Faculty of Dental Surgery (MFDS). The dental graduate will then be required to obtain a medical degree and, in practice, a place would not be given in a medical school without the attainment of the MFDS examination. The would-be surgeon should make every effort to obtain a place in one of the available shortened courses (three to five years) to prevent training becoming unduly long and arduous. The dental graduate has been given a dispensation to sit the part I MRCS exam during the medical preregistration year and once in possession of both the MFDS and the MRCS he or she may then enter a specialist five-year training programme approved by the Specialist Advisory Committee in Oral and Maxillofacial Surgery.

Maxillofacial surgery is not for the faint-hearted because of the long training programme and the highly specialized nature of the work, but the rewards are high. The maxillofacial surgeon deals with referrals from both dental and medical practitioners for conditions involving the mouth, jaws and dental structures but also more far-reaching problems such as conditions of the salivary glands and head and neck oncology, and currently 80% of oral cancers in the UK are treated by maxillofacial surgeons. Much satisfaction is gained in the surgical management of congenital and acquired deformities of the face and jaws such as cleft lip and palate. Increasing collaboration with neurosurgery, not only for facial deformity and facial fractures but also access surgery for cranial lesions, is an exciting new development. The maxillofacial surgeon is additionally now responsible for the management of the majority of facial injuries.

The pathway for the student who undertakes medicine first is very similar, with a dental qualification being obtained during a shortened undergraduate dental course. The dental graduate, however, has the advantage that before undertaking this arduous training programme they have already established an affinity for this type of work during their dental undergraduate education.

Myth	A bunch of dentists practising surgery.
Reality	Highly motivated, well-qualified surgeons practising anatomically based surgery in the head and neck area. An expanding surgical spectrum consequent on dual qualification in both medicine and dentistry and a well defined training programme.
Personality	Outgoing, energetic, plenty of stamina, a thick skin and a high degree of manual dexterity.
Best aspects	The visual nature of work in the head and neck area is technically very demanding but good results are achieved in the majority of patients.
Worst aspects	Long and arduous training programme.
Requirements	MFDS, FRCS(OMFS) in addition to both a medical and dental degree.

Hours

Junior   Consultant

Numbers 260 posts   0.5% are women.

Competitiveness

Stress

On-calls

Junior   Consultant

Salary

£50 000   £90 000   £350 000

For further information

British Association of Oral and Maxillofacial Surgeons
Royal College of Surgeons of England
35–43 Lincoln's Inn Fields
London WC2A 3PN
Tel: 020 7405 8074
Fax: 020 7430 9997
Website: www.baoms.org.uk

Plastic and reconstructive surgery

Plastic surgery is a small specialty in terms of numbers of consultant posts and, perhaps for this reason, even one's hospital colleagues are not entirely sure what one does. It is, therefore, helpful for anyone considering plastic surgery as a career, not to wear a pinstripe suit or a bow tie but to have a small element of paranoia in his personality!

The specialty is concerned with restoration of form and function to as near normality as possible. It overlaps with many other surgical specialties, plastic surgeons often providing soft tissue cover and repair at these interfaces: for instance, trauma and orthopaedic surgery in the care of upper or lower limb trauma cases, maxillofacial and ENT surgery in head and neck cancer and general and breast surgery in breast reconstruction. The care of burns involves interaction with intensive care specialists and skin oncology dovetails with dermatology. Cleft lip and palate surgery is a truly multidisciplinary activity.

Because of the small number of training and consultant posts, there is fierce competition to get on to a training scheme. Within the MRCS a basic surgical rotation which includes plastic surgery would give an opportunity for a leg-up when applying for higher surgical training schemes. Useful specialties to have covered in basic surgical training would be orthopaedics, general surgery and any of neurosurgery, ENT or paediatric surgery. As yet, the Calman scheme is not smoothly moving from basic surgical training to higher surgical training without some holding step to gain more experience and improve the CV prior to an HST Appointments Committee, but once the bottle-neck is cleared, it is then a conveyor belt of six years to full accreditation and sitting the FRCS(Plast) examination. Research is a rewarding ingredient of the higher surgical training timetable and the opportunities here are enormous. Subjects include studies on the microcirculation, nerve regeneration and repair, skin substitutes, the study of skin tumours and transplantation biology.

There is no such thing as a routine reconstructive procedure and worldwide literature in reconstructive surgery is ever changing so that new ideas from around the world need to be assimilated, criticized, adopted or abandoned. Refinements in methods of 'stealing' tissue from one part and transferring them to another, while minimizing the donor site defect, are constantly appearing in the scientific journals or being reported at meetings.

Just as the plastic surgeon needs to understand the patient's problems in the context of his/her own surgical abilities, the patient also needs to have realistic expectations of the outcome. This is particularly so in the field of aesthetic surgery (also known as cosmetic surgery) which is largely practised outside the NHS but whose techniques are employed all the time for NHS patients, such as in the attention to detail in the repair of a cleft lip.

Those plastic surgeons who wish to work their evenings and weekends can generate money at a rate slightly less than their families can spend it, but not everyone chooses to climb on this treadmill. A happy balance between technical satisfaction and financial reward can be found in this small but evolving specialty.

I seem to have got a bit carried away with the reconstruction, but I'm sure it will come in useful...

Myth	A bunch of smoothies running around shovelling bucket-loads of silicone into the rich and brainless.
Reality	A creative subspecialty with foundations in basic surgical sciences where a large armamentarium of surgical techniques enables creative and artistic restoration of function and form.
Personality	An ability to understand sensitively and discuss patients' problems and offer realistic expectations of reconstructive outcomes, perhaps staged over several years. Self-critical perfectionists with a hint of paranoia commonly apply.
Best aspects	Satisfaction for the patient and the surgeon can result from a short local anaesthetic procedure or a long microsurgical procedure. Often patients become friends of the surgeon as their surgery and follow up can be prolonged.
Worst aspects	Disappointment when complicated techniques fail, thereby losing the best reconstructive option. There is a growing culture of medicolegal complaints which may result in a lesser reconstruction being offered since some 'Rolls Royce' results require risks.
Requirements	FRCS(Plast) MS, MD etc. do not go amiss.

Hours

🕐 🕐 🕐 🕐 🕐   🕐 🕐 🕐 🕐 🕐

Junior   Consultant

Numbers   228 posts, 10–12 per year   12 are women

Competitiveness   🗡 🗡 🗡 🗡 🗡

Stress   ☹ ☹ ☹ ☹ ☹

On-calls

📟 📟 📟 📟 📟   📟 📟 📟 📟 📟

Junior   **Consultant** can be variable but
                                         consultant-requiring
                                         emergencies are common

Salary

£min   £av   £max

£50 000   £90 000   £500 000

For further information	**British Association of Plastic Surgeons** Royal College of Surgeons of England 35–43 Lincoln's Inn Fields London WC2A 3PN Tel: 020 7831 5161/2 Fax: 020 7831 4041 Website: www.baps.co.uk

Hand surgery

The hand has a great many intricate mechanisms in a confined and vulnerable area and the management of the whole spectrum of hand problems demands skills which are part of both orthopaedic and plastic surgery. Hand surgery has grown as a specialty since World War II. In the 1960s the British Society for Surgery of the Hand was established and has since fostered the specialty.

Hand surgery is still firmly rooted in the orthopaedic and plastic surgery specialties and in order to train as a hand surgeon it is necessary to proceed through one of these pathways. At present, consultant posts are still advertised for orthopaedic or plastic surgeons with an interest in hand surgery. However, by the time a student now interested in hand surgery reaches that stage it is likely that pure hand surgery posts will be appointed since replacements will be needed for retiring surgeons who have moved towards 100% hand surgery and also because there is a major move throughout Europe and beyond to establish a separate specialty.

Most trainees start with an interest in orthopaedic or plastic surgery and gravitate towards the hand. Hand disorders can, to some extent, be divided between the two disciplines, although many patients have problems that cross over the boundary. Therefore, it is essential that the hand surgeon should have at least some experience in the other discipline. It is intended that candidates should cross from one to the other specialty for this advanced training. Under the Calman unified training programme, a year of hand training would most likely be held in year 5.

Qualifications for the practice of hand surgery are those of the parent specialties. An academic degree such as an MD or MS is an asset but not essential. A European diploma is available on examination to suitably qualified surgeons who have completed training (the first sitting was in 1996).

Hand surgery has a diversity demanding a high degree of technical skill combined in some areas with diagnostic facility and some knowledge of other disciplines including rheumatology, neurology, rehabilitation, paediatrics and, of course, orthopaedic and plastic surgery with their basic sciences. The spectrum of work encompassed by a hand surgeon who crosses the orthopaedic surgery/plastic surgery divide includes:

- acute trauma of all the various tissues extending up the limb;
- reconstruction after trauma to skin, tendons, bone, nerves (including tendon transfers) and blood vessels; and acute and chronic trauma reconstruction which may require microvascular techniques;
- congenital malformations of the hand and upper limb;
- rheumatoid and osteoarthritis;
- neurological disorders such as cerebral palsy and the effects of quadriplegia;
- tumours, benign and malignant;
- miscellaneous disorders such as Dupuytren's disease and tendon entrapments like trigger finger.

Technical and research challenges abound in hand surgery and advances are taking place in microvascular reconstructive surgery and peripheral nerve surgery, including the treatment of nerve root avulsion from the spinal cord. Steady progress is also being made in the understanding of tendon healing and the nature of Dupuytren's disease. Finally, refinements in surgical technique are constantly being introduced.

Myth	How can anyone focus on such a limited anatomical field?
Reality	A broad and complex anatomical area involving much of the upper limb. It is the most commonly injured part of the body and one of the most vital to most occupations. After the face, it also carries the most aesthetic significance.
Personality	Technically motivated; prepared to treat trauma out of hours.
Best aspects	Fascinating range of work. Rewarding to restore function. Technical challenges. Possible to do much work under local anaesthetic and therefore independent.
Worst aspects	If patients are not motivated even good operations cannot work.
Requirements	FRCS, FRCSOrth. or Plast.

Hours

Junior   Consultant

Numbers   20 exclusive posts   190 ortho/plastic posts with a strong interest

Competitiveness

Stress

On-calls

Junior   Consultant

Salary

£50 000   £90 000   £150 000

For further information	**British Society for Surgery of the Hand** Royal College of Surgeons of England 35–43 Lincoln's Inn Fields London WC2A 3PN Tel: 020 7831 5161 Fax: 020 7831 4041 Website: www.bssh.ac.uk

Neurosurgery

Although trepanning of the skull was practised in Stone Age times, it is only in the past 100 years that surgery of the central nervous system has been practised with any reasonable prospect of a good result. In the early days, surgery was usually performed on patients during the late stages of brain compression from tumours and blood clots so death after surgery was a common event. Nowadays, with better anaesthesia, control of intracranial pressure, operating microscopes and pre-operative imaging and intraoperative computer guidance, removal of tiny abnormalities deep within the brain is possible and relatively safe. However, mishaps still occur all too readily and anybody contemplating a career in neurosurgery must have plenty of stamina as the work is long and demanding, and have the psychological make-up that will question in depth the causes of a disaster but not be unduly depressed by it. Strong self-belief is important, often misinterpreted as excessive ego. A commonly heard comment is 'The only difference between God and a neurosurgeon is that God doesn't think he is a neurosurgeon'. (Many neurosurgeons would see that as one of God's failings!)

It would be wise to include a neurosurgical SHO post during basic surgical training to test the water as in-depth exposure to the specialty as a student is rare. After MRCS the six-year higher neurosurgical training consists of five years in clinical neurosurgery and one year of options, involving research, subspecialty interests or overseas experience. Nowadays most neurosurgeons will be looking for consultant posts in their mid-thirties, 10–15 years after qualifying. There has been a considerable increase in the number of neurosurgeons in the last few years, driven by subspecialization and the need to have more surgeons covering these subspecialties. While there are still a few small centres where general neurosurgery is covered by three or four neurosurgeons the major centres will now have between six and ten surgeons. The major subspecialties are vascular, spinal, paediatric, oncological, pain and functional. Some rare disorders are still treated at supraregional centres, such as paediatric craniofacial surgery for which there are only four centres in the country.

Neurosurgery is a consultant-led service and the recommended caseload for an individual neurosurgeon according to the Society of British Neurological Surgeons is about 250 cases per year. The case mix is changing rapidly. Spinal surgery is drifting towards neurosurgeons and away from orthopaedic surgeons, although in some centres a new hybrid spinal surgeon has emerged with training in both disciplines. Conversely vascular neurosurgery is drifting towards the interventional neuroradiologist leaving the vascular neurosurgeon to deal with the difficult aneurysms the radiologists cannot treat.

Technology is impacting more on the neurosurgeon. Nowadays instead of looking at CT or MRI scans and working out in your mind where the lesion is and assessing the best approach a computer will do this for you giving a 3-D reconstruction of the patient's head and directing a route to the lesion avoiding unfriendly structures. Endoscopy is used to treat some forms of hydrocephalus and open magnets allow the possibility of perioperative MRI scanning with patient and surgeon in the magnet. However, the surgeon still needs good hand–eye co-ordination whether using clever toys or not.

Myth	Clever egotists whose patients all end up as cabbages.
Reality	Clever egotists, some of whose patients end up as cabbages but most don't.
Personality	Dextrous psychopaths who can be very analytical when problems occur but appear emotionally unaffected by them.
Best aspects	Fascinating work. Once people realize you are not joking when you say you are a brain surgeon you gain instant social credibility.
Worst aspects	Long hours, even as consultant.
Requirements	FRCS(SN)

Hours

Junior   Consultant

Numbers   160 posts   6–8 per year   5% women

Competitiveness

Stress

On-calls

Junior   Consultant

Salary

£50 000   £110 000   £400 000

For further information

Royal College of Surgeons of England
35–43 Lincoln's Inn Fields
London WC2A 3PN
Tel: 020 7405 3474
Fax: 020 7831 9438

Society of British Neurological Surgeons
Website: www.eans.org

Orthopaedic surgery

Orthopaedic surgery encompasses the management of fractures and trauma as well as management of degenerate disorders of bones and joints. The majority of orthopaedic surgeons have responsibilities for the supervision and treatment of trauma patients for part of their working week and for the remainder will run elective clinics and operating lists. Some centres have specialized trauma units, just like *ER*!

Advances in the management of trauma care have occurred particularly in the last 20–30 years and many fractures are now treated operatively rather than conservatively. The fracture is returned to as near an anatomical position as possible and is then held in place with the use of metal plates, nails or external fixation frames. This more aggressive approach is particularly appropriate in younger patients or where many injuries have occurred (polytrauma). The orthopaedic surgeon works in conjunction with accident and emergency departments, plastic surgeons and general surgeons in the management of these problems.

In the area of elective surgery tremendous changes have occurred due to the increasing use of joint replacement surgery and minimally invasive surgery of joints. Joint replacement first began in the early 1960s and now accounts for a large part of the workload of an orthopaedic surgeon. Nearly 100 000 joint replacements are performed per annum in the UK and 5% of people aged over 65 will have had a hip replacement. Arthroscopic and minimally invasive surgery is used more commonly and it is likely that early intervention with these techniques in arthritic joints will be possible. Surgeons specializing in minimally invasive surgery often have an interest in the management of sports injuries particularly of the knee and shoulder.

Traditional areas of orthopaedic interest include paediatric disorders and spinal disorders. Surgeons in these areas are often highly subspecialized. A further area of subinterest is surgery of the hand which is covered separately.

The specialist registrar posts are limited and the competition is correspondingly great. The training is six years of which a minimum of three and a half years must be spent in clinical practice before taking the exit (FRCSOrth) examination. The other years are spent in research or flexible attachments, which allows the development of an interest in, say, hip or shoulder surgery. Some orthopaedic surgeons will not pass through the specialist registrar posts but will become clinical lecturers, posts which are funded by the university and allow accreditation in orthopaedic surgery but with greater emphasis on research.

There is relatively little requirement for treatment of cancer and life-threatening conditions and the emphasis is very much on improving quality of life and diminishing disability. There is tremendous scope within orthopaedics for further advances in surgical techniques and the specialty is likely to continue expanding over the next 10–20 years. As increasing numbers of people participate in sporting activities this area of work will expand and an increasing elderly population will mean there is more and more requirement for joint replacement surgery.

Myth	Male rugby-playing sportsmen three times as strong as an ox and half as bright.
Reality	Increasing numbers of women now go into orthopaedic surgery. There is much greater emphasis on academic achievement and much orthopaedic surgery requires fairly fine motor skills attracting people with an interest in microsurgery and minimally invasive surgery.
Personality	Encompasses a wide range of personality types. Some will require little sleep and live on adrenaline spending their time managing major trauma cases. Others will be interested in sports injuries and drive fast cars. Some will be interested in management of children and drive old Morris Minors.
Best aspects	Busy, satisfying job with tremendous variety during the working week. Tremendous range of operations to perform and types of patients to treat. The majority of orthopaedic procedures are performed for non-life-threatening conditions and result in decreased pain and disability in patients. As a result patients are generally very satisfied and grateful.
Worst aspects	Busy workload with high-pressure clinics and long waiting lists. Trauma work can involve a considerable amount of out-of-hours commitment.
Requirements	FRCS(Orth)
Hours	Junior ●●●●○ Consultant ●●●●○
Numbers	1200 posts only 12 women
Competitiveness	▼▼▼▽▽
Stress	☹☹☹☺☺
On-calls	Junior ●●●●○ Consultant ●●●○○
Salary	£min £50 000 £av £100 000 £max £400 000
For further information	**British Orthopaedic Association** Royal College of Surgeons of England 35–43 Lincoln's Inn Fields London WC2A 3PN Tel: 020 7405 6507 Fax: 020 7831 2676 Website: www.boa.ac.uk

Trauma surgery

Trauma surgery is a wildly exciting specialty especially when you are young. In a major disaster you are the key player, and in the polytraumatized patient with horrendous injuries and blood everywhere you are in charge. If that is not enough, you have the most beautiful Meccano sets in the world ready in an operating theatre purpose-built for reconstructing human bodies. What more could you want?

Many of your patients are young, keen on sport and fun to work with so why isn't everybody doing trauma surgery? Well for a start there are, as yet, very few trauma surgeons. Most of this work is supervised by general orthopaedic surgeons who spend the rest of their time doing elective orthopaedics (e.g. hip replacements and other routine operations).

The major problem with trauma is that the hours are very irregular. You never know when the next major accident will come in. There is either too little work or far too much. Operations can last over 12 hours and may start at any time of the day or night. Big units could plan things so as to reduce this disruption but there are very few units in Britain large enough to manage this.

The key to the job is decision-making ability and leadership. Clinical decisions have to be taken at very short notice, often with inadequate information. You probably need to be fairly thick-skinned to live with the fact that inevitably some of your decisions will prove to have been wrong in retrospect. This surgery is never routine. Each injury has its own particular problems and solutions. Being able to conceptualize in three dimensions and be a lateral thinker probably helps. As you get older the attractions of being a front-line doctor with all these diverse skills may get tempered by the desire for a little order in your life at work and at home. Trauma surgery cannot be tailored to a comfortable 9-to-5, five-days-a-week job.

The training is as for any orthopaedic surgeon, continuing up to the exit examination, FRCS(Orth). A one-year fellowship abroad in a country with a more violent lifestyle (e.g. USA, Canada or South Africa) will be useful. Currently, there are far more consultant jobs being advertised in orthopaedics and trauma (over 150 each year) than there are trainees (a mere 60 each year) so you can afford to be selective. Trauma surgery does not have much private practice compared with elective orthopaedics, but there is scope to supplement your salary by writing medical reports for patients who are involved in litigation after the accident. There is a huge demand for this type of mundane work at the moment, so you never need starve.

Like many of the acute specialties this job may appear very attractive to a doctor starting out but there are not quiet pastures here for those peaceful years when the fires of ambition and the craving for excitement have burned down to the embers of a good night's sleep and reasonable salary. This career is not for the faint-hearted.

Myth	Lantern-jawed, strong as an ox, able to operate for long periods completely submerged in blood.
Reality	A new specialty for Britain, offered as a major subspecialty interest by most consultants when applying for a job that they want—dropped with equal alacrity by the same consultants as a specialty interest as soon as they have been appointed.
Personality	Obsessional workaholic, lives on adrenaline, adores expensive and technically complicated gadgets and then hits them with a hammer.
Best aspects	Very exciting. If there is a disaster you are it (in fact you probably caused the disaster). You don't spend much time in outpatients. There is room for an almost infinite expansion of your salary by performing rather dreary medical reports for personal injury.
Worst aspects	The hours can be appalling, most major accidents occur late in the afternoon or through the night. There is no private practice. Anaesthetists avoid you (your lists are, by definition, unplanned). Burn-out: trauma may be fun when you were young but as you get older . . .
Requirements	FRCS(Orth)

Hours

Junior: four and a half clocks   Consultant: five clocks

Numbers — 1500 ortho/plastic posts, most with a trauma interest   25 women

Competitiveness — five scalpels

Stress — five unhappy faces

On-calls

Junior: four and a half pagers   Consultant: four pagers

Salary		
£min	£av	£max
£50 000	£80 000	£150 000

For further information	Consultants in a trauma centre, or: Royal College of Surgeons of England 35–43 Lincoln's Inn Fields London WC2A 3PN Tel: 020 7405 3474 Fax: 020 7831 9438 Website: www.boa.ac.uk

Paediatric surgery

Paediatric surgery is divided into general paediatric surgery and specialist paediatric surgery. Although much general paediatric surgery is performed in district general hospitals by adult surgeons, specialist paediatric surgery is confined to regional centres. In most centres there are five or more specialist paediatric surgeons of whom one will be a paediatric urologist. Currently it is recommended that there is one specialist paediatric surgeon per 500 000 population.

Historically surgeons have moved into the speciality of paediatric surgery during a training in general surgery. Although this still occurs to some extent, trainees are increasingly entering the speciality at an earlier stage and are encouraged to gain experience in paediatric or neonatal medicine. Specialist registrars are appointed to a training programme in one of six training consortia in the UK and Ireland and will be expected to rotate through at least two of the consortium centres during the six-year training programme.

Paediatric surgeons work very closely with their paediatric medical colleagues and in most centres have a far closer working relationship with paediatricians than they do with other surgical specialities. The surgery comprises a number of areas of major surgery. Neonatal surgery includes the management of congenital defects such as oesophageal atresia, congenital diaphragmatic hernia, abdominal wall defects and intestinal obstruction. These patients require complex treatment and subsequent follow-up throughout childhood. Many neonatal conditions are now diagnosed on prenatal ultrasound and thus there are close working relationships between paediatric surgeons and fetal medicine specialists. Increasingly there is a role for the surgeon in prenatal counselling.

In addition to neonatal surgery all centres are involved in major gastrointestinal surgery, the surgery of solid tumours of children, and paediatric urology. In some centres paediatric surgeons will also perform thoracic surgery (but not cardiac surgery).

Paediatric surgery is immensely rewarding. Children tend to recover very quickly, even from major surgery, and are less prone to complications. Fortunately deaths are very rare but there are particular stresses involved in managing sick children and their parents. The informality inherent in paediatrics results in a relaxed and open approach to patient care. It is difficult to indulge in pompous pontification on a ward round with a two year old trying to pull your trousers down!

In addition to the specialist paediatric surgeon outlined above, the role and training of general surgeons who undertake surgery on children in district hopitals is becoming better defined. In the past surgeons have undertaken this role without formal training. The current recommendation is that such surgery should only be performed by designated surgeons who have received at least six months' training in a specialist paediatric surgery centre. It is therefore possible for a general surgeons to consider developing a subspeciality interest in paediatric surgery during general surgery training.

Myth	A weird group of surgeons whose practice is confined to circumcisions.
Reality	One of the bastions of 'general' surgery. Many paediatric surgeons undertake a wide range of gastrointestinal surgery and some thoracic, plastic surgery and neurosurgery; a significant proportion of the work is urology. The specialty is expanding rapidly with close links to paediatric medicine.
Personality	Should enjoy working with children and their parents and enjoy the challenge of technically demanding surgery.
Best aspects	Broad range of surgery. Good training scheme. An evolving surgical specialty with considerable overlap with other specialties.
Worst aspects	Emotional stresses of dealing with sick children and their parents. Heavy out-of-hours workload.
Requirements	FRCS(Paediatrics)

Hours

Junior   Consultant

Numbers   85 in total   4% are women   2 or 3 qualify per year

Competitiveness

Stress

On-calls

Junior   Consultant

Salary

£50 000   £60 000   £100 000

For further information	**British Association of Paediatric Surgeons** Royal College of Surgeons of Edinburgh 35/43 Lincoln's Inn Fields London WC2A 3PN Tel: 020 7869 6915 Fax: 020 7869 6919 E-mail: adminsec@baps.org.uk Website: www.baps.org.uk

Transplantation surgery

The first successful transplant was performed in Boston in 1954 between identical twins. In Britain, transplantation started in the early 1960s and became an established form of renal replacement by the 1970s, with one-year graft survival rates averaging 69–70%. Now, good units are achieving greater than 90% one-year survival rates.

Transplantation surgery offers an intellectually stimulating career. It is an area of clinical expertise which demands working alongside physicians.

- **Kidney transplantation** takes place in 23 centres throughout the UK each performing between 50 and 140 transplants per year. Each unit should be staffed by four consultant surgeons most of whom will have a second speciality interest such as urology, endocrine surgery or vascular surgery (access surgery for haemodialysis forms the major part of the work of most renal transplant surgeons). The number of kidney transplants being performed in the UK is stable (about 1700 per year of which approximately 10% are performed from living donors). There are serious consultant staff shortages in most units; there are currently 15 consultant vacancies based on the number of existing kidney transplant units.

- **Liver transplantation** is performed in seven centres which are all based at major teaching hospitals and which also provide the staff for abdominal organ transplant retrievable throughout the UK. Techniques are evolving to enable small children to be transplanted with fragments of liver from adult cadaveric donors or from living related donors. Although there is some staffing shortage it is not as severe as with kidney transplantation, but based on current work patterns two new consultant liver transplant surgical posts need to be filled each year.

- **Heart and lung transplantation** is carried out in five centres. The incidence of heart disease in the UK is enormous but the number of heart transplants done is relatively small and totally dependent on suitable organ donors.

- **Pancreatic transplantation** which is well established in the USA has not been popular in the UK although the development of islet transplantation would appear to be a satisfactory way to encourage uptake. Small intestinal transplantation is performed only sporadically and remains near experimental.

The training for abdominal organ transplantation depends upon the career intention of the individual. A career in kidney transplantation with a second specialty is common. Six-year training programmes are currently being developed which will include two years of kidney transplantation included in the five/six years of either vascular, general or urology training. Training in liver transplantation is highly specialized and such surgeons usually have training in upper intestinal surgery and other forms of liver surgery.

The need for high-quality transplant surgeons has never been greater. It is unlikely that this form of surgery will become outmoded such as other areas of technology which have changed the nature of clinical practice beyond recognition.

Myth	Body-snatchers, workaholics, love operating in the middle of the night.
Reality	A career for the thinking surgeon, incorporating intensive patient care, general medicine, nephrology, immunology and some psychology. Not for the 'cut-and-run' surgeon.
Personality	Mainly committed workaholics.
Best aspects	Holistic approach to patient care, integrated surgical and medical care, interesting surgical and medical problems. Giving patients a new lease of life—tangible results with grateful patients.
Worst aspects	Small units. Many consultants on continuous call or one in three, often with non-specialist juniors. Being seen as mere technicians at the beck and call of nephrologists. Little or no private practice.
Requirements	FRCS, MS or MD useful

Hours

Junior · Consultant

Numbers 118 posts 18 per year (often unfilled) four women only

Competitiveness

Stress

On-calls

Junior · Consultant

Salary

£60 000   £80 000   £100 000

For further information	**Chairman of the Training Committee** British Transplantation Society Triangle House Broom Hill Road London SW18 4HX Tel: 020 8875 2430 Fax: 020 8875 2421 E-mail: secretariat@bts.org.uk (Catriona Sanderson) Website: www.bts.org.uk

Urology

Urological surgery involves the investigation and treatment of surgically correctable conditions involving the genitourinary system which implies cooperation with specialists in renal medicine and gynaecology; as many urological conditions are amenable to medical treatments, consulting and diagnostic skills are required in addition to surgical aptitude. Because the whole of the urinary tract is amenable to direct inspection endoscopic diagnosis and surgery are fundamental to the practice of urology. Since many endoscopic surgical procedures are conducted solely using a television monitor, spatial awareness and perception are both important.

Subspecialization in urology is commonplace and urologists often develop areas of particular expertise within their more general urological practices. Some urologists specialize in the surgical treatment of malignant diseases of the urinary tract. Prostate cancer is increasing worldwide and diagnosis and treatment of this condition are occupying more of urologists' caseloads. Subspecialization also includes urogynaecology with particular reference to treatment of urinary incontinence and the practice of andrology, which deals with the treatment of functional and physical disorders of the male genitalia including male infertility. The treatment of urinary tract stone disease is often considered a subspecialty particularly in centres using shockwave-generating machines (lithotripters) to disintegrate urinary stones without the need for surgery. Renal transplantation is often performed by urologists who have undergone subspecialty training.

Urology is an acute specialty involving daily emergency admissions such as urinary retention, urinary tract infections and renal colic, but most of the urgent operations can be fitted into normal working hours which has much appeal.

Urological training proceeds as with other areas of specialist surgery and the six-year training programme is supervised by the Specialist Advisory Committee in Urology at the Royal College of Surgeons. After a minimum three-year period of core training and success at the FRCS(Urol) exam come opportunities for subspecialist training. The specialist exam itself reflects the range of urology and covers the following topics: oncology; stone disease and infections; trauma, female urology and dysfunction; paediatric urology; nephrology, including transplantation and basic science; benign prostatic hypertrophy, andrology and bladder reconstruction.

Myth	Sensible surgeons who deal with incontinence.
Reality	A rapidly expanding surgical specialty now regarded as separate from surgery in general. Urologists are trained to operate via the endoscope but also enjoy a range of open urological procedures. The development of innovative technology has been rapid in this specialty and there is scope for the development of televisual and robotic procedures.
Personality	Varied, ranging from the oncological surgeon, via the minimally invasive to the innovative technologist.
Best aspects	Well-organized training scheme. A cohesive and happy group of specialist surgeons whose subspecialist interests allow continued personal development even at consultant level. Minimal out-of-hours operating commitment.
Worst aspects	Demand for urological services still outweighs supply and therefore there is tremendous pressure to treat more patients, particularly in respect to the very heavy outpatient workload compared with in-patient bed availability.
Requirements	FRCS(Urol)

Hours

Junior ⏰⏰ Consultant ⏰⏰

Numbers 500 posts (25 per year) 10% are women

Competitiveness 🗡🗡🗡

Stress ☹☹☹

On-calls

Junior Consultant

Salary

£min £av £max

£50 000 £80 000 £250 000

For further information	**British Association of Urological Surgeons** Royal College of Surgeons of England 35–43 Lincoln's Inn Fields London WC2A 3PN Tel: 020 7405 1390 Fax: 020 7404 5048 Website: www.baus.org.uk

Vascular surgery

This specialty has blossomed over the past 30 years both in terms of volume and technical advances. As a result there has been a rapid expansion in the number of vascular surgery posts and the demand for consultants in this specialty continues to increase. In most hospitals vascular surgeons continue their involvement in the acute general surgical workload so that some vascular surgeons are pure specialists while others may spend half of their time on other general surgical procedures. This allows flexibility for the trainee who may be interested in the subject but is uncertain whether he or she wishes to be a pure specialist.

The surgery is complex and demanding with a premium on technical skill. Another major characteristic of the specialty is the very close association with other specialties, such as interventional radiology, cardiology, cardiac surgery, renal and diabetic medicine. For those interested in the subject this allows for fruitful discussion and an increased understanding of the widespread nature of arterial disease. Thus, the vascular surgeon finds himself or herself involved with a wide variety of problems in diverse anatomical sites, carotid disease, thoracic outlet problems, visceral and renal ischaemia, aneurysms and, increasingly, demanding distal revascularization in the legs. The surgeon will also frequently be asked his or her opinion on circulatory problems that do not require surgical intervention, such as Raynaud's disease, scleroderma, deep venous thrombosis and pulmonary embolism.

Vascular surgery is an important part of acute general surgery and the close interaction with other surgical colleagues adds further breadth to the job. Training comes under the umbrella of surgery in general with two years of basic surgical training (BST). For those interested in becoming vascular surgeons it is prudent to 'test the water' with a six-month BST attachment to a vascular unit but this, of course, is not imperative. The upper levels of higher surgical training can be obtained on a busy vascular unit with all the facilities and the specialist registrar should obtain good exposure to the majority of vascular procedures before obtaining the CCST. At this point he or she is in a position to apply for a consultant post but may wish to spend a year as a vascular Fellow in order to obtain further experience in more complex surgery. In the final FRCS examination the vascular trainee can request a viva in vascular surgery but the examination remains the test for surgery in general. The European Board of Vascular Surgery was formed in 1995 and began examining for a European qualification in vascular surgery in 1996.

Vascular surgery is a demanding and exacting specialty and one of the most rapidly changing fields as technology advances. Also, as life expectancy improves, patient expectations particularly in terms of quality of life are increasing and atherosclerosis is endemic: there is quite a future for the vascular surgeon.

Myth	The interventional radiologist will take over and amputation remains inevitable.
Reality	Technical advances and an increasing awareness of the disease are leading to an ever-expanding necessity for intervention. This requires harmonious cooperation between radiologists and surgeons, and despite the fact that percutaneous vascular intervention has been practised for 30 years the demand for vascular surgery continues to increase.
Personality	Calm under pressure. A lot of stamina and enthusiasm.
Best aspects	Complex and demanding surgery with a premium on technical skill. The satisfaction of successfully managing a patient through the procedure by judicious control of cardiac and renal functioning, etc. Close and long-term care of patients. The training goals are well defined. This specialty requires commitment since much of the management is urgent or emergency.
Worst aspects	Arterial reconstructions are unforgiving of technical errors and there can be stressful moments when, for example, haemorrhages are difficult to control.
Requirements	FRCS

Hours

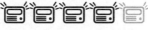

Junior   Consultant

Numbers   580 posts   1% are women

Competitiveness

Stress

On-calls

Junior   Consultant

Salary

£50 000   £100 000   £200 000

For further information

Royal College of Surgeons of England
35–43 Lincoln's Inn Fields
London WC2A 3PN
Tel: 020 7973 0306
Fax: 020 7430 9235

CHAPTER 3

Reproductive health

Obstetrics and gynaecology

General training

Most undergraduates find their midwifery experience very appealing but when they start their specialist training wonder why they chose a specialty that gets them out of bed so much! Obstetrics and gynaecology maintains its attraction however, because of the diverse range of clinical disciplines and opportunities dealing with relatively young patients whose medical problems have added emotional and social aspects. Obstetrics and gynaecology remained an essentially surgical specialty until about 25 years ago. Whilst it has now blossomed into several distinct subspecialties most consultants still train as generalists, usually with a subspecialty interest. All obstetricians and gynaecologists must combine knowledge of physiology, endocrinology, sexuality, pharmacology, pathology, neonatology, general medicine and surgery with their specialized skills.

Within obstetrics comes the challenge of the physiological changes of pregnancy, which affect every organ system of the body, complicate the management of concurrent diseases and modify the effects of medications. Basic practice ranges from antenatal care, as a critical exercise in preventive medicine, to the skills of instrumental delivery of babies, backed up by the modern management of physical and biochemical disorders of the fetus.

Gynaecology also offers diversity. Macroscopic, microscopic and endoscopic surgical skills are needed in the treatment of genital cancers, prolapse, urinary incontinence, menstrual disorders and infertility. Medical skills are required in the treatment of endocrine and other disorders, amenorrhoea, infertility, recurrent miscarriage, hirsutism, menstrual pubertal and postmenopausal problems, as well as in everyday contraception. Sexual dysfunction may come into every aspect of practice and requires special sensitivity.

Training starts at SHO grade for one or two years, closely supervised by a consultant and specialist registrar. Trainees usually also spend a year, or two periods of six months, in associated specialties such as neonatal paediatrics, anaesthetics, gastrointestinal or urological surgery, endocrinology or gynaecological pathology. This is usually at SHO grade but may be later during specialist registrar training, before the fourth year.

MRCOG Part I in basic sciences is needed for entry into a specialist registrar training scheme. Research training for at least one year is encouraged and is usually fitted in before the fourth year. A research degree is usually necessary to be competitive for later subspecialty or academic training.

The first three years as a specialist registrar are in general obstetrics and gynaecology. The final Part II MRCOG is best taken in this time. For general training, the extra two years involve more exposure to the subspecialties, providing an opportunity to develop a special clinical interest for the future in consultant practice. Generalist or special interest specialist registrar training is for five years to reach the CCST or six years for subspecialists. In addition certified accreditation in specialist techniques such as colposcopy, ultrasound and minimal access surgery is becoming mandatory for continuing practice. All specialist registrars, whether generalists or subspecialists, have attended training courses relevant to their practice on audit, epidemiology, ethical and legal issues, medical administration, NHS and general management, risk management and statistics.

Nationally there are currently 1026 recognized specialist registrar posts. There have recently been considerable problems for trained specialist registrars as a result of a slowing down of the previous

Obstetrics and gynaecology: career pathway

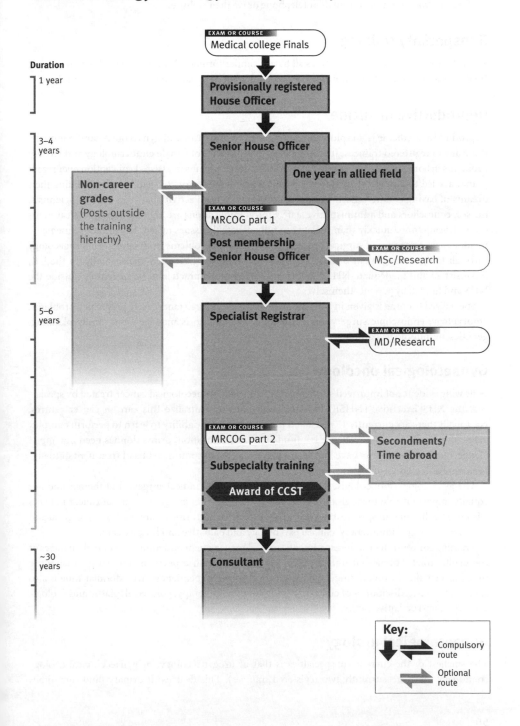

Duration

1 year

3–4 years

5–6 years

~30 years

EXAM OR COURSE
Medical college Finals

Provisionally registered House Officer

Senior House Officer

One year in allied field

EXAM OR COURSE
MRCOG part 1

Non-career grades
(Posts outside the training hierachy)

Post membership Senior House Officer

EXAM OR COURSE
MSc/Research

Specialist Registrar

EXAM OR COURSE
MD/Research

EXAM OR COURSE
MRCOG part 2

Secondments/ Time abroad

Subspecialty training

Award of CCST

Consultant

Key:

Compulsory route

Optional route

high rate of consultant expansion, but all this is likely to change: it is worth checking with the Royal College of Gynaecologists by e-mail or telephone or via their website.

Subspecialty training

The subspecialty training programmes all have a similar format. This is of a period of two years of (usually modular) clinical training and (at least) one year of research relevant to the subspecialty.

Reproductive medicine

Reproductive medicine is a rapidly developing area of obstetrics and gynaecology, and nationally there are 15 registered trainees. It encompasses many aspects of female endocrinology and fertility problems in both females and males. Extraordinary developments in assisted conception over recent years have led to a range of treatment options which help doctors to help couples fulfilling their dreams of having children. Each assisted conception is a team activity between doctors, scientists, nurses, counsellors and administrative staff. Ethical implications are enormous as new treatments often develop more quickly than society can fully debate the issues raised. Reproductive medicine includes a diverse range of surgical procedures and medical problems from adolescent gynaecology through to the management of hormonal problems following the menopause. Sadly, in the UK, inconsistent and inadequate NHS funding has forced much practice to be in centres outside the NHS and funded by patients themselves.

Specialized training is given in conception physiology and assistance, early pregnancy problems, embryology, endoscopic surgery, endocrinology, endometriosis management, family planning, genetics, immunology, pathology and pharmacology.

Gynaecological oncology

Following evidence of improved survival of patients with gynaecological cancer treated by specialists, the NHS Executive (NHSE) has approved plans to centralize this care in cancer centres. Nationally there are currently 17 registered trainees. Whilst the ability to learn to perform complex surgical procedures with excellence is a fundamental qualification, prima donnas need not apply! Gynaecological oncologists have to be team players, as the optimum results of treatment of malignancy are obtained through team care.

The gynaecological oncologist does of course perform the radical surgery, but there is another equally important role through the coordination and the assessment and care of cancer patients with team colleagues in specialist nursing, diagnostic imaging, critical care, pathology, clinical and medical oncology, radiotherapy, clinical psychology and palliative and hospice care.

Training concentrates on the assessment, surgical management and follow-up of malignancies of the genital tract. Specialized training is also given in relevant aspects of colposcopy, diagnostic imaging, genetics, histopathology, intensive care and high dependency care. Modular time is also spent in the allied disciplines of clinical oncology and radiotherapy, colorectal, plastic and urological surgery and palliative care.

Gynaecological urology

The smallest of the current subspecialties is that of urogynaecology, or gynaecological urology (nationally there are currently two registered trainees). This deals with urinary (and sometimes faecal) incontinence as well as genital prolapse. Most senior gynaecologists have spent many years dealing with prolapse and incontinence during their careers and some believe that urogynaecology is just part of general gynaecology. However, recent research and understanding of the mechanisms of this distressing condition have challenged this view.

There are currently only a few recognized centres for subspecialty training in urogynaecology, and probably only a small increase in number is required to produce the correct number of uro-gynaecological subspecialists needed for the UK. The trained urogynaecological subspecialist may find limited job opportunities, as few trusts require this level of expertise, which is currently only available on a regional or supraregional basis.

Maternal and fetal medicine

This involves the highly clinical specialized care of two patients: mother and fetus. For subspecialist care, mother, fetus or both must have a pathology which requires expert judgement in diagnosis, counselling and treatment. This field is constantly evolving as innovative new therapies are considered, tested and introduced. Nationally there are currently 26 registered trainees.

Maternal medicine covers management of conditions coexistent with pregnancy as well as conditions that arise secondary to pregnancy, such as pre-eclampsia, HELLP syndrome and thromboembolism. It predominantly involves antenatal assessment and management, but can lead to emergency care of seriously ill women in the delivery suite, which can easily be seen as an ITU.

Fetal medicine, in contrast, focuses on developmental problems and their early recognition. It includes prenatal diagnosis of genetic, chromosomal and structural abnormalities and the diagnosis, management and treatment of pathological conditions such as fetal anaemia, disturbance of growth and problems related to multiple pregnancy. Ultrasound is a major tool, used to complement diagnosis, investigation and treatment. There is no room for a shaky hand—an exacting technique is required for sampling a moving target! Counselling skill is also an important requirement for example, in relation to continuing the pregnancy with an expected poor outcome for the baby or terminating the pregnancy.

The maternal/fetal medicine specialist coordinates the care for the remainder of the pregnancy and delivery, involving team work between medical, midwifery and support staff as well as with the major paediatric subspecialties who will take over the care of the neonate after birth.

Specialized training is given in imaging and associated invasive investigations and treatments. Relevant aspects of fetal anatomy, embryology, physiology and pathology are also covered together with maternal physiology, pathology and pharmacology. Modular time will also be spent in ultrasound, neonatal paediatrics and genetics.

Community gynaecology

Community gynaecology is the most recent subspecialty to be recognized. Nationally there are currently six registered trainees. The role of the community gynaecologist is still evolving and differs around the country. All consultants have responsibility for the management of women's healthcare in the community, together with associated training and research and will supervise provision of and training in family planning. Most will also have a coordinating role in sexual healthcare—genital cancer screening, abortion and sterilization services, liaison with social and other services, youth advisory work, prevention of genitourinary infection and management of certain gynaecological problems such as premenstrual and menopausal symptoms.

Specialized training is given in management and administration, contraception, management of unwanted pregnancy, health screening, climacteric and medical gynaecology management and psychosexual and forensic sexual management. Modular time is also spent in colposcopy, genito-urinary medicine and public health medicine.

Myth	Attracts types who like or dislike women too much and become smooth owners of villas in Little Venice.
Reality	Whilst there are rewarding private practices in every part of the country you have to learn to cope in training and as a consultant with strenuous night work. The range of clinical and intellectual interests provides the main satisfaction.
Personality	Empathic, with varied interests from *in vitro* fertilization research types to more traditional surgeons. Can be particularly charming.
Best aspects	Patients relatively young and alert with strong emotional and social elements adding appeal to all aspects of practice. Private practice plentiful and rewarding.
Worst aspects	Night work. Heavy routine workload due to rapid development of the specialty not matched by consultant numbers. Current severe mismatch between number of CCST holders and consultant vacancies has recently resulted in a reduction in recruitment of specialist registrars.
Requirements	MR COG and second degree, especially in MD, as this is usually needed for choice posts.

Hours

🕐🕐🕐🕐🕐   🕐🕐🕐🕐🕐

Junior   Consultant

Numbers 1200 posts   9% increase per year   20% are women.

Competitiveness 🗡️ 🗡️ 🗡️ 🗡️ 🗡️

Stress ☹️ ☹️ ☹️ ☹️ ☹️

On call

Junior   Consultant   Private obstetrics
(maximum allowed) (shared NHS rota)

Salary

£min   £av   £max

Consultant: £50 000   £100 000   £300 000

For further information	Royal College of Obstetricians and Gynaecologists 27 Sussex Place Regent's Park London NW1 4RG Tel: 020 7772 6200 Fax: 020 7207 723 0575 E-mail: coll.sec@rcog.org.uk Website: www.repromed.net and www.rcog.org.uk

Family planning and reproductive healthcare

In an over-populated world, family planning and reproductive healthcare are crucial links in the chain of health and arguably represent one of the most important areas of medical practice. In most developed countries, contraceptive services are provided by hospital gynaecologists, but in some, including the UK, the needs of most patients are provided through primary care.

Family planning is now part of the core curriculum of the MRCGP qualification, as well as being a syllabus requirement for MRCOG and required experience for those entering genitourinary medicine. However, those doctors working in the community family planning clinics provide specialist contraceptive services and the bulk of theoretical and practical training in family planning. Working in this service requires, at a minimum, the Diploma of the Faculty of Family Planning and Reproductive Health Care at the Royal College of Obstetricians and Gynaecologists (DFFP of the FFPRHC of the RCOG). Many prospective GPs, gynaecologists, genitourinary medicine physicians, and others, take this diploma as a means of acquiring a recognized recertifiable qualification in family planning.

Training consists of a theoretical component, usually covered in a two-day programme of lectures and workshops, which is followed by supervised clinical training. The DFFP can often be taken in evening courses, thus allowing it to be taken in parallel with other training. Additional training is offered in intrauterine techniques and subdermal implants, as well as postgraduate education, for those wishing to become recognized as family planning instructing doctors. Doctors who have undergone this type of training work as clinical medical officers (CMOs) and senior clinical medical officers (SCMOs).

In a departure from higher training programmes leading to attainment of consultant status, the FFPRHC of the RCOG has now instituted a three-year career-grade training programme. This training is designed to produce lead SCMOs functioning at subconsultant level. The pilot centres have already been taking people through this programme and a transition year will be advertised for year 2000, during which the Faculty will give out its own career-grade training numbers. A prerequisite for this training is that the trainee should have completed two years of basic medical experience including evidence of gynaecological experience equivalent to that obtained during a six-month post in combined obstetrics and gynaecology. Entry requirements include passing Part I MFFP or Part I MRCOG. At the end of training, the Faculty will ratify completion of training and issue the trainee with a certificate confirming such completion. Whilst this certificate will not be recognized as a legitimate qualification under GMC or European Community rules, it will serve to confirm that the trainee has undergone a structured training programme recognized by a duly constituted Faculty of a Royal College. It will confirm that the trainee has the relevant experience and expertise to take up a post with responsibility for leading a service or part of a service in family planning and reproductive healthcare (SCMO or associate specialist).

Note, as in the previous section in obstetrics and gynaecology that, within the new subspecialty of community gynaecology, family planning and reproductive healthcare play a large part.

Myth	Failed obstetricians and gynaecologists, non-academic middle-aged female part-timers in sensible shoes.
Reality	A rapidly expanding new 'specialty' almost unique to Britain which has a major role to play in attaining and maintaining high standards of reproductive healthcare. Family planning *per se* remains unrecognized as a specialty in its own right but community gynaecology is currently offered as a subspecialty of obstetrics and gynaecology.
Personality	Varies, but all are highly motivated. Inter-active skills are of prime importance at all levels, not just with patients, but also for team building.
Best aspects	Ability to improve standards of care in reproductive health and female reproductive and sexual health in particular.
Worst aspects	In spite of rapid expansion, and overall importance, it is still considered a 'Cinderella' speciality. However, changes are afoot to accord it its rightful place.
Requirements	MFFP and MRCOG if operating skills required. MRCOG a must for subspecialists in community gynaecology and reproductive health.

Hours

Junior   Consultant

Numbers 66 posts (consultant community gynaecologists or consultants in family planning and reproductive healthcare or other titles) of which women occupy 60.

Competitiveness

Stress

On-calls

Junior   Community-based   Hospital-based
         consultants   consultants

Salary

£47 000   £54 000   £62 000

For further information	**Subspecialty Training Committee** Royal College of Obstetricians & Gynaecologists 27 Sussex Place London NW1 4RG Tel: 020 7772 6200 Fax: 020 7723 0575	For career-grade training: **Faculty of Family Planning and Reproductive Healthcare of the RCOG** 19 Cornwall Terrace London NW1 4QP Tel: 020 7935 7162 Fax: 020 7935 8613

CHAPTER 4
Anaesthetics

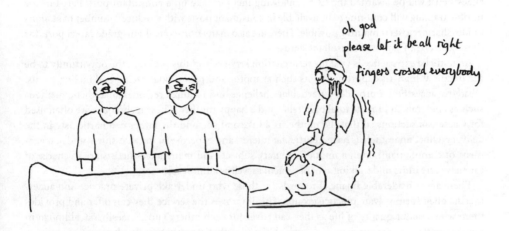

oh god
please let it be all right

fingers crossed everybody

Overview

Anaesthetics is a very popular specialty; indeed, it has more consultants than any other. The increasing use of local and regional as well as general anaesthesia has increased the scope of anaesthesia for surgery. Anaesthetists are also involved in the relief of post-operative, obstetric and chronic pain, as well as intensive care medicine. Many anaesthetists subspecialize in these areas or have a particular interest in anaesthesia for specialist surgery such as paediatric, cardiothoracic, neurosurgical, plastic and burns surgery, or orthopaedic surgery.

All anaesthetists in the UK are qualified doctors who undertake a six-year structured training programme. The first two are in the SHO grade, learning the basic science and practice of anaesthesia and pain control; during this period the trainee will usually pass Primary FRCA. They are then eligible to enter the specialist registrar grade for five years of training. By the end of the first registrar year they should have passed the final part of the FRCA examination. There is the opportunity to gain specialized training and to do research during the last years of training after which the anaesthetist will be awarded the CCST, allowing them to take up a consultant post. Part-time or flexible training will continue to be available in consultant posts with a reduced number of sessions or job-sharing posts remaining possible. There are also many non-consultant-grade career posts for those who do not aspire to consultant status.

Anaesthetic experience is vital for resuscitation services and this provides the opportunity to be the doctor at high-risk sporting events such as motor and power boat racing and boxing events. Obstetric anaesthetics provides a particular challenge and requires regional anaesthetic methods such as epidurals to provide total pain relief and a happy mother. These techniques are often used for Caesarean sections so that the mother is awake and she and the father can participate in the delivery. Other anaesthetists have a particular interest and expertise in the assessment and management of chronic pain, often a multidisciplinary subject, and many anaesthetists are in charge of intensive care units undertaking a management as well as clinical role.

There are considerable financial rewards for those who undertake private practice and anaesthetists often form private practice groups. This improves the service they can offer and provides them with a better quality of life as they can cover for each other. Thus, anaesthesia, although in many respects a service specialty and in which the anaesthetist works very much as part of a team, is very rewarding and the results are usually immediate and very apparent. The ability to relieve pain also gives enormous satisfaction.

The FRCA examination

This is a two-part examination. The first part can be sat after gaining 12 months' experience in anaesthesia and consists of a paper with 90 multiple-choice questions (MCQ), an OSCE and two half-hour viva examinations. It covers basic sciences, clinical anaesthesia and pharmacology. The second part can be sat after 36 months' experience. It consists of a 90-question MCQ paper, a 12-question, three-hour short answer paper and two half-hour vivas. It covers the same ground in more detail as well as medicine and surgery as applied to anaesthesia. It also covers intensive care and chronic pain management.

Anaesthetics: career pathway

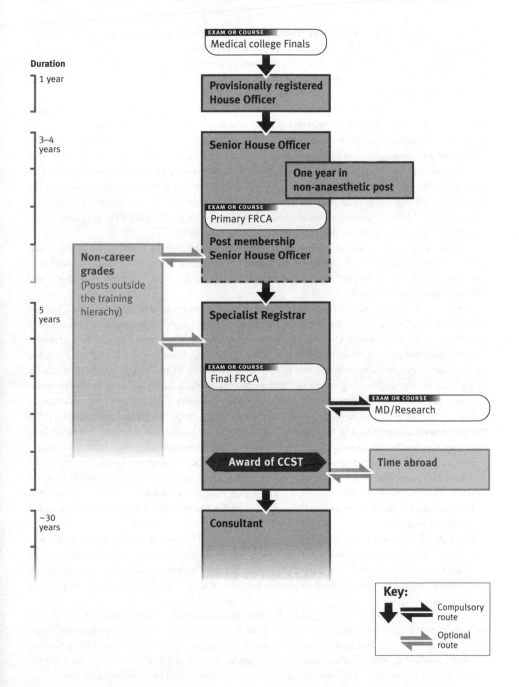

Duration

1 year

3–4 years

5 years

~30 years

EXAM OR COURSE
Medical college Finals

Provisionally registered House Officer

Senior House Officer

One year in non-anaesthetic post

EXAM OR COURSE
Primary FRCA

Post membership Senior House Officer

Non-career grades
(Posts outside the training hierachy)

Specialist Registrar

EXAM OR COURSE
Final FRCA

EXAM OR COURSE
MD/Research

Award of CCST

Time abroad

Consultant

Key:

Compulsory route

Optional route

Anaesthetics

The main activity of the majority of anaesthetists is the safe management of anaesthesia for operative and allied procedures. This begins at the pre-anaesthetic visit, which is normally carried out the day before operation, in the case of in-patient surgery. However, with the increasing tendency to admit patients on the day of surgery, and therefore the need to carry out the assessment on the same day, the anaesthetist often has a very early start to his/her day.

The average pre-anaesthetic assessment takes about 15 minutes, but this may extend to a much longer period if there are special problems of a physical or psychological nature. The latter is fairly common and includes concerns on the part of the patient: that (s)he may not be adequately asleep for the surgery, may not come safely through the anaesthetic and surgery, may experience undue post-operative pain or may suffer post-operative nausea and vomiting. It is the anaesthetist's duty to reassure the patient in these regards and to grade the patient's anaesthetic. After assessment the anaesthetist advises the patient in outline of the nature of the anaesthetic, whether it be general, regional, local block or 'sedonanalgesia'. Also advised is the degree of pain that the patient may reasonably expect to experience and the methods of relief available.

With the array of drugs and techniques available today, it can truly be said that 'there is no such person as an unanaesthetizable patient', although the anaesthetist will need to assess the degree of risk inherent in the anaesthetic against the complexity and urgency of the required surgery and advise the patient accordingly.

During administration of the anaesthetic, the anaesthetist will be assisted by a dedicated, trained 'anaesthetic assistant': an operating department assistant (ODA), operating department practitioner (ODP) or an anaesthetic nurse. Often there are trainees in anaesthesia, trainee ODAs, ODPs or anaesthetic nurses, and medical students doing their anaesthetics attachment. Sometimes there are other professionals who are there to be trained in specific procedures. These include ambulance officers doing their 'paramedic' training and nurse trainees and midwives. It is a challenge to be able to maintain safe anaesthesia for a patient and at the same time provide training and guidance to such trainees.

During the preoperative period, the anaesthetist not only keeps the patient pain-free but also monitors all vital functions. The most important of these is the integrity of the brain, but since there is no practical method of directly observing cerebral activity under general anaesthesia, the anaesthetic challenge is to ensure brain integrity by ensuring adequate patient ventilation (whether it be spontaneous or artificial), adequate cardiac output and oxygenation and effective removal of carbon dioxide. All this is now possible with the technological methods available for patient monitoring, but it must always be remembered that the anaesthetist is the patient's monitor and all so-called monitors are mere aids.

The duty of the anaesthetist to his/her patient extends well beyond the preoperative phase and into the period of post-anaesthetic recovery, which is nowadays carried out in a dedicated recovery ward adjacent to theatres and may even extend to the patient's own (surgical) ward. Aspects of such care include postoperative pain relief, fluid and electrolyte balance and the provision of anti-emetic therapy.

Anaesthesia is the clinical specialty which has the greatest diversity of interests and activities, not only in terms of interests outside the operating room, such as obstetrics, acute and chronic pain relief and intensive care, but also within anaesthetics itself. It is now possible to specialize in cardiac, thoracic, paediatric, orthopaedic, vascular, ophthalmic, maxillofacial, ENT anaesthesia, etc.; the variety is quite remarkable. The anaesthetist's life is now a rich, varied and rewarding one.

Myth	Bored doctors doing *The Times* crossword with a patient on autopilot. The 'brain' side of the blood–brain barrier.
Reality	A dynamic expanding specialty with a wide variety of fascinating patient care. Involvements in anaesthesia have facilitated the expansion of surgery so that no part of the body is inaccessible and no operation too major to contemplate.
Personality	Varied; ranges from the ITU physicist to the laid-back surfer.
Best aspects	Dealing with all aspects of medicine. The results are immediately apparent. There is enormous personal satisfaction in the relief of pain and in providing life support to the critically ill.
Worst aspects	Occasional sheer, blind terror; the status quo can change very quickly. Contribution not always recognized by patients and medical colleagues. Having to deal with the vanity of many surgeons.
Requirements	FRCA (and MD for academic posts).

Hours

Junior   Consultant

Numbers   2500 posts (200 per year)   25% are women

Competitiveness

Stress

On-calls

Junior   Consultant

Salary

£50 000   £75 000   £200 000

For further information	**Royal College of Anaesthetists** 48–49 Russell Square London WC1B 4JY Tel: 020 7813 1900 Fax: 020 7813 1875 Website: www.rcoa.ac.uk

Intensive care

Intensive care medicine is arguably the most specialized area of medicine of all. The intensive therapy unit (ITU) is a specialized area of the hospital, with dedicated staff, characterized by one-to-one nursing and very high levels of medical involvement in patient care. The sickest patients, character-ized by failure of at least one organ system, are cared for on the ITU. Failure of the respiratory system, requiring ventilation, can only be managed in the ITU. Therefore, the most common route into ITU training is via anaesthetics. It is also possible to train in ITU from other backgrounds, but these routes are complex (see below). All anaesthetic rotations will involve a period of intensive care, at SHO as well as specialist registrar levels. This helps fulfil a service commitment to the unit, as well as giving experience in ITU to the doctors.

ITU nurses are usually much more highly trained than most. They are familiar with all aspects of their patient's care and can consequently seem intimidating at first, but are usually fiercely loyal. ITUs are rarely quiet. The government is currently looking to expand the number of beds in most areas. In the meantime, most units remain at near capacity, or full, for the majority of the time. As a consequence of this, and the fact that the patients are far sicker than those in the rest of the hospital, ITU is a very busy speciality for all levels of staff.

The successful ITU physician needs to be prepared to work long hours, to be called at short notice and to have to make decisions quickly. Whilst all aspects of the patients' physiology can be manipu-lated, modern technology cannot save a patient from multi-system organ failure, and the ability to let go is a requirement of the job. Communication skills are understandably vital, liaising with anxious relatives and explaining care to other teams within the hospital in a non-antagonistic way as well as working with the dedicated multidisciplinary team on the unit itself.

Training

The current proposals for entry to and completion of a programme of training leading to a CCST in intensive care medicine (ICM) are as follows. The CCST in ICM will consist of SHO and specialist registrar training, the content of each being the same for trainees entering from all specialties. Entry to specialist registar training in ICM will require the trainee to have satisfactorily completed SHO training including not less than six months' medicine, six months' anaesthesia and six months' ICM training (in blocks of not less than a month); then to have first been successfully appointed to a substantive specialist registrar post in a parent speciality and hold an NTN and then to have been competitively appointed at a later date to an approved specialist registrar training programme in ICM.

The specialist registrar training in ICM will comprise six months' training in approved posts at intermediate level in blocks of not less than three months as described by the Intercollegiate Board for Training in Intensive Care Medicine (ICBTICM) and 12 months' training in approved posts at advanced level. The CCST in ICM will only be awarded after successful completion of training in the parent specialty.

Competitive entry into the specialist registrar grade in ICM training will be via two routes, either directly off existing anaesthetic rotations or competitively for those joining from other specialties. In all other respects the entry criteria and training programmes will be identical and will be moni-tored by the ICBTICM.

Myth	Over-cerebral gasmen who say no too frequently and prolong the inevitable.
Reality	A multidisciplinary specialty involving the sickest patients in the hospital. Extremely hard pressed and hard worked; whilst most things are possible, miracles are hard to achieve.
Personality	Varied, with room for all types, though thick skinned and pragmatic with a scientific inclination may be an advantage. Good communication skills essential
Best aspects	Intensive care medicine embraces the most modern and invasive of technologies and works hand-in-hand with highly experienced and motivated nurses and professionals allied to medicine. Saving the very sickest patients in the hospital; having some of the best resources at your disposal.
Worst aspects	Colleagues and the general public have increasingly unrealistic expectations of what intensive care medicine can achieve. A proportion of intensive care patients die despite all efforts. Shortfalls in the delivery of critical care tend to be drawn into the political spotlight on a seasonal basis.
Requirements	FRCA, MRCP, FRCS (and MD for academic posts)
Hours	Junior Consultant
Numbers	900 not all are pure intensivists
Competitiveness	
Stress	
On-calls	Junior Consultant
Salary	£50 000 £65 000 £90 000
For further information	**Intensive Care Society** Tavistock House Tavistock Square London WC1H 9HR Tel: 020 7631 8890 Fax: 020 7631 8897 E-mail: admin@ics.ac.uk Website: http://www.ics.ac.uk	**Royal College of Anaesthetists** 48–49 Russell Square London WC1B 4JY Tel: 020 7813 1900 Fax: 020 7813 1875 Website: www.rcoa.ac.uk

Pain management

Pain management is a new and expanding area of interest for anaesthetists. In the early days anaesthetists were called upon by clinicians to utilize their practical skills to perform nerve blocks for patients with cancer-related pain. From this developed a much greater interest in the management of all patients with chronic or intractable pain. Most large hospitals now provide some facility for pain management though so far it is largely an untapped market.

The development of Acute Pain Services in the 1980s has also expanded so that there is a natural progression from the perioperative period to those unfortunate patients who go on to sustain long-term pain and disability. The subject is extensive and today a wide range of conditions are treated from the control of low back pain, to the management of cancer and to the understanding and control of pain from nerve injury (neuropathic pain). The traditional interest for anaesthetists has been the employment of practical skills performing injections and other invasive procedures. However, it is now recognized that a much greater component of the work involves getting to grips with the behaviour of patients and identifying *why* they should develop pain rather than just how it happens. For the majority, finding a cure for their condition is an unrealistic goal and a more practical approach is to encourage techniques and treatment strategies that offer patients the ability to cope more effectively with their pain.

Most clinicians involved in pain management work as part of a team, which may involve psychologists, occupational therapists, complementary therapy specialists and physiotherapists. Pain management is still recognized as a subspeciality within anaesthesia. Anaesthetists going into pain management need to be good communicators and have considerable tolerance and an ability to cope with unhappy, and sometimes difficult, people. The subject offers a good opportunity to practice clinical pharmacology and to interact with patients more effectively than in other situations.

Doctors usually become interested in pain management once they have started on a formal anaesthetic training programme. During the specialist registrar years trainees are often exposed to patients who suffer chronic pain and also have the opportunity to deal on the wards with the routine issues related to postoperative pain management. Before completion of training they will have been expected to attend the chronic pain management facility for at least three months. This, of course, is insufficient for anyone wishing to pursue a career in pain management and inevitably following the completion of training it is expected that doctors will spend a further period of six months or more further developing their skills.

During the training module, it will be expected that skills will be developed in the practical procedures, in counselling, in the use of complementary treatments and in the appropriate management of patients through medication.

Within the UK there are very few posts which are solely devoted to pain management and most Health Authorities advertise pain management posts in conjunction with some anaesthetic commitment.

Chronic pain management is a consultant-run service and whilst some centres may offer in-patient facilities the majority of doctors would practice the speciality on an out-patient or day-patient basis. Although it is necessary to provide a continuous service, it is likewise recognized that most chronic pain problems are rarely 'emergencies' in the true sense of the word and problems late at night are fairly infrequent. However, the work is demanding and the hours are often long.

Myth	Part-time anaesthetists pushing pills at the neurotic.
Reality	Now recognized as a speciality. Multidisciplinary approach involving a wide variery of modes of treatment from drugs to behavioural therapy.
Personality	Empathic and tolerant with a good scientific understanding. Communication skills essential.
Best aspects	Good one-to-one interaction with patients; a very broad range of options to choose from including complementary therapies. Improving the quality of life of people who thought they would never be free of pain.
Worst aspects	Some extremely demanding, dependent or neurotic patients. Some patients remain in pain.
Requirements	Currently FRCA possibly MRCP.

Hours

Junior   Consultant

Numbers   around 100 posts

Competitiveness

Stress

On-calls

Junior   Consultant

Salary

£min   £av   £max

£50 000   £70 000   £120 000

For further information

Royal College of Anaesthetists
48–49 Russell Square
London WC1B 4JY
Tel: 020 7813 1900
Fax: 020 7813 1875
Website: www.rcoa.ac.uk

CHAPTER 5

General practice

Overview

General practice is now called primary healthcare (hospital being secondary heathcare, and referral from one hospital department to another being tertiary heathcare). To satisfy political efforts to make the NHS financially viable, the GP is now, as well as being a generalist in professional terms, a small businessman, a member of a financial syndicate, responsible to both the government and to the individual for 24 hour care of the people of this country. The GP is still, however, the family doctor, and this role remains one of the most satisfying in medicine. General practice is regarded by many specialists as the most demanding job of the lot, covering as it does the full spectrum of ill health from the cradle to the grave, for some 2000 people per doctor. No other field provides such total patient care. General practice attracts many of the best graduates, who can, even in these cynical times, enjoy a particular relationship with people and a unique professional challenge.

While few set out to be GPs, about half of medical graduates become GPs. GPs are usually self-employed, although under the authority of the Health Authority which controls their budget. Most work in partnerships, with a team of their own choosing, they employ office and nursing staff—more behind the scenes than is generally realized. Lay managers may be employed leaving the doctors free to do the clinical work. At least one partner should have a feeling for finance; those practices that have not yet coalesced into Primary Care Trusts are paid by a complex system of claims and allowances, so that efficient book-keeping is essential.

Practices vary from establishments like mini hospitals, where partners specialize, to single-handers, and from inner-city groups with multicultural changing populations, to Herriot-type rural practices where winter visits are made on a tractor or pony. Partnerships recruit members whose interests differ from their own, ensuring a well rounded team. Women are well represented, many now choosing salaried posts allowing them increased mobility. Salaried doctors on short-term appointments cover some of the most difficult areas in city centres.

Each practice is responsible for the health of the patients registered with it for 24 hours a day. This is the area of greatest change within a generation, as out-of-hours demand has increased beyond the emergency provision originally envisaged. The availability of local rotas to share this responsibility is of great importance to the wellbeing of the GP.

The following accounts indicate the range of styles of practice styles. The enthusiasm for the job remains clear.

General practice: career pathway

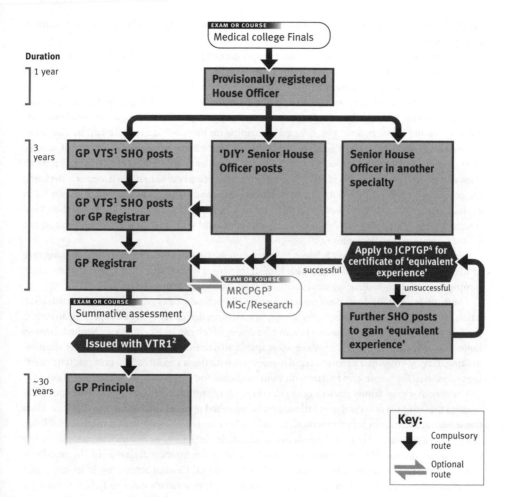

Duration

1 year

3 years

~30 years

EXAM OR COURSE
Medical college Finals

Provisionally registered House Officer

GP VTS[1] SHO posts

'DIY' Senior House Officer posts

Senior House Officer in another specialty

GP VTS[1] SHO posts or GP Registrar

GP Registrar

Apply to JCPTGP[4] for certificate of 'equivalent experience'

successful

unsuccessful

EXAM OR COURSE
MRCPGP[3]
MSc/Research

EXAM OR COURSE
Summative assessment

Issued with VTR1[2]

Further SHO posts to gain 'equivalent experience'

GP Principle

Key:

↓ Compulsory route

⇨ Optional route

Approved Specialties for GP Training

- General medicine
- Geriatric medicine
- Psychiatry
- Paediatrics
- General surgery
- Accident and Emergency medicine (or A&E with either surgery or orthopaedics)
- Obstetrics and/or Gynaecology

Further guidance in the JCPTGP booklet 'Guide to Certification'.

Notes

1 GP VTS – General Practice Vocational Training Scheme.

2 VTR1 is the form signed by GP trainer after successful completion of the final training year.

3 MRCPGP = Membership of the Royal College of General Practitioners (an exam based diploma.)

4 JCPTGP is the Joint Committee on Postgraduate Training for General Practice, 14 Princes Gate, London SW7 1PU.

General practice

People have an advocate in their GP who does not stand to gain by the advice given; this state of affairs is almost unique to Britain.

About 90% of medical consultations take place in general practice. The GP is the doctor who sees the patient first, facing the challenge of diagnosis. The ill must be distinguished from the worried well, the few requiring specialist attention from those—the vast majority—whose care can be provided within the practice. Hospital consultants see patients only after filtering through primary care. This system protects the patient from unnecessary or repetitive investigation, and husbands hospital resources. Patients may be referred to hospital for investigation to establish the diagnosis, for treatment such as surgery only available in hospital or for advice on problems of disease management. It is of great importance to listen to the patients' underlying concerns, to establish trust and rapport and maybe to explain to a patient why a second opinion is not necessary. Resisting unrealistic expectations is part of the job, as is being open to criticism. Equally it may be helpful to explain that medicine is not an exact science and that judgement is involved. GPs know their local consultant specialist colleagues, their particular interests and skills and their personalities, and can advise patients in their best interests.

When the hospital teams have achieved all they can, the patient comes home to the ongoing care of his or her GP, who enables those with long-term illness to live with their disease, monitoring symptom control, co-ordinating care, accessing services and validating claims.

There are snags: long hard days under pressure (50 patients a day when busy); the frustration when resources are limited, of patients having to wait for relief; never being an expert on anything; the responsibility for staff, i.e. having to run a business, which can be fun for some; limited income; huge amounts of imposed change; the inescapable malaise of inner cities; and lonely decision making. Having congenial partners, regular meetings with them and attending postgraduate meetings—essential for keeping up to date with both medicine and community—relieves isolation.

The special joys of family doctoring are the ongoing relationships, knowing the wider ramifications of the family over several generations and being called upon as a trusted friend. Patients often come with problems not strictly medical, including life events and social and emotional problems. Good management of birth and death are particularly satisfying, as is enabling people to live with chronic disease. Just as rewarding is the buzz of an unexpected diagnosis in the middle of morning surgery, or saving a life in the middle of the night. Clinical autonomy is an important aspect of this branch of medicine, as is facilitating the patient to have a voice and choice whenever possible. GPs are the last generalists, increasingly filling a vacuum left by greater specialization in the hospitals.

Leading people through episodes of illness or anxiety with kindness and competence is rewarding. The family doctor is a confidential, approachable professional who can be relied upon for unprejudiced advice, practical help and ongoing interest and concern. The general surgeons and physicians of old are dying breeds, which leaves a real need for those with a full toolbox.

Myth	Kind chaps in tweeds who couldn't make consultant and spend their afternoons on the golf course
Reality	Large numbers of women. Practical generalists. The gatekeepers of the NHS working as the patient's advocate. Small businessmen with an immensely satisfying way of life.
Personality	Empathic, conscientious, pragmatic, kind; have genuine liking for people. Omnivorous interests.
Best aspects	Autonomy, variety, responsibility for the whole patient acting as the patient's advocate. Satisfying long-term relationships with patients of all ages. Opportunities for part-time work or salaried work.
Worst aspects	Overload by fallout from cost-cutting and secondary care. Twenty-four-hour responsibility without the manpower to provide a shift system. Being stuck with tiresome patients.
Requirements	See training diagram (MRCGP useful)

Hours

rural   inner city

Numbers	35 620 posts; 30% are women (55% of registrars)
Competitiveness	none

Stress

On-calls

rural   (or deputizing)
                            inner city

Salary

£30 000   £52 000   £80 000

For further information	**Royal College of General Practitioners** 14 Prince's Gate London SW7 1PU Tel: 020 7581 3232 Fax: 020 7225 3047 Website: www.rcgp.org.uk

Academic general practice

Some would say this is the ultimate oxymoron! Yet all over the world, academic general practice (known in the USA as family practice) is developing. This former cottage industry of medicine is gaining a firm foothold within universities and medical schools.

Academic general practice is the study of, and teaching about, general practice. It often happens in universities but anyone working in or near general practice can get involved. General practice needs its own body of specialized knowledge and expertise, established through GP-based research.

Medical students find that learning is great fun in the informal setting of general practice. They learn much basic medicine with one-to-one teaching and friendly feedback, and also learn about primary care itself, where most illness episodes are dealt with in their entirety.

While general practice, in the form of a community-based personal medical service, is very old, academic general practice has developed almost entirely within the last 50 years. The College of General Practitioners was founded in 1952 and the first GP professor in the world took up his chair in 1963.

The tension between academic life and the pragmatic individualism of general practice has made it a slow business to get a clear academic career pathway. It is clear that good training in research and teaching methods, with real projects, with students and with close supervision are essential to long-term success. There will always be a difficult balance between gaining enough experience and training in active general practice and timing one's entry into the world of academia.

There is no fixed career pathway for this field but recommendations include gaining academic experience early (a BSc, especially in primary care, epidemiology, sociology, anthropology, psychology or management of economics). Ensure one's training jobs are stimulating, give a broad range of experience and encourage independent thought. Membership of the Royal College of General Practitioners (via the membership exam) is essential for a career in academic general practice and one should try to join one of the junior academic training fellowships. It is of course important to work for two or three years in a busy practice to gain a proper perspective on what is important to patients.

Academic general practice suffers from academic and bureaucratic inertia, multiple commitments, endless funding applications, constant committees, and less money than purely clinical practice. However, it provides a tremendous variety of research opportunities. It allows one to test out ideas, to teach (at all levels) and to try to change the world for the better!

Inner city practice—a personal view

Working as a GP in central London has been the most challenging experience of my medical career. I work in a typical inner city area characterized by extreme contrasts. Most patients are healthy but some are ill; many are poor and unemployed; a few are wealthy. 'No go' housing estates sprawl out along the high street, not far from fine Victorian villas, set back in landscaped gardens. Corner shops and overcrowded launderettes stand beside some of the most expensive antique shops in England. Restaurants catering to the cuisines of a dozen different countries line the streets leading to nearby theatres but thin out quickly in the vicinity of bed-and-breakfast hostels and refugee centres.

With patients originating from over 30 different countries the practice as a whole is aware of many family and social networks, local housing developments and local political issues. We maintain close contact with street agencies, welfare rights organizations, social workers and patient groups. A 'wealth of living pathologies' daily poses a variety of clinical challenges certainly as hard, and sometimes as rare, as any to be expected in finals. Surgeries usually last three hours and involve listening, touching, talking, examining, investigating, monitoring, treating and referring people. A consultation that may involve a highly structured and somewhat ritualized clinical assessment of a complex disease, such as diabetes, may be immediately followed by another in which I need to rely upon my intuition and judgement. General practice medicine demands mental acrobatics and jack-in-the-box techniques not often taught in medical school.

Ethical dilemmas are common and continuing. Can I get an extra contractual referral organized for a patient without breaching confidentiality? How can I find out whether the patient sitting before me knows what I know about her partner's hepatitis B carrier status? A few patients are seriously ill and dying, some with intractable pain, who clearly possess sufficient medication to commit suicide if they so choose. With such a high percentage of unplanned pregnancies 20% of pregnant patients in our practice request abortions annually. I finish with an intravenous opiate addict, requesting injectable methadone; I ponder how to weigh his words about 'staying out of trouble'.

As self-employed practitioners, we GPs have chosen to work together. We employ our own staff which allows us a degree of control over our working practice and over the ethos and ambience of the practice (rare anywhere else within the NHS).

In London, because of competition from better paid jobs outside the health service, choice of staff is frequently restricted. Nevertheless, I believe that those who work in general practice have many more opportunities than most to develop and to practise their own distinctive style of healthcare.

GPs who practise in inner cities undoubtedly work in poorer circumstances than most other family doctors and are relatively less well remunerated. But they are rewarded by close contact with a panoply of differing peoples, of diverse traditions and cultures, and with varied healthcare problems. In tackling many of the health issues that arise in these often dislocated communities, we participate in and gain much from the richness and complexity of inner city life.

Remote rural general practice

Remote rural general practice is about working in a close-knit community. It allows you to raise your children in a safe and healthy environment. There is a shortage of doctors willing to work in rural practice despite the obvious attractions and the efforts made in recruitment. One possible reason for the recruitment problems is thought to be that school pupils from rural areas have a lower chance of being accepted in medical schools through achieving slightly lower grades than those from urban schools and are interviewed by a selection committee composed of hospital consultants with a limited perspective. Another is that this way of life does not suit everyone and both practitioner and partner must want to be in this environment.

There are increasing opportunities for students and junior doctors to spend some time in a rural practice without having to commit themselves. In Scotland and Australia for example, rural doctors talk about their work through seminars and lectures in schools and some medical schools arrange for undergraduates to have their GP training within a rural practice.

The World Organization of National Colleges Academique of Family Practice (WONCA) is supporting recruitment programmes for doctors in remote rural areas and has published a paper for relevant medical educational and training bodies.

For very isolated practitioners, the NHS gives special help in two ways (detailed in *A Statement of Fees and Allowances Payable to General Practitioners in England and Wales* (the 'Red Book'):

(1) *The inducement scheme:* where there is a very small list, the health authority provides a surgery and house for the doctor and guarantees a net income which is 80% of the national average.

(2) *The associate scheme*: this was introduced in 1990 to provide the finance to enable a young doctor to be employed between two or three isolated practices, which not only enables the associate to gain special experience but gives intermittent relief for the practitioners themselves.

Most young graduates entering general practice join a local scheme which gives them two years of training through approved hospital posts and a year in a training practice all within the same area. During that time, some of them have the opportunity to exchange with a trainee in a rural practice. However, it is not essential to join a scheme, and by planning their own series of posts, trainees have the opportunity to experience hospital posts in different parts of the country as well as working for six months or a full year in an isolated training practice.

Once training for general practice has been completed, whether it be in a rural or city practice, and the certificate from the Joint Committee for General Practice Training has been obtained a post as an associate practitioner can be sought. In addition, there are numerous openings through locum work, in order to 'test the water' in an isolated practice and see if you would enjoy the swim.

With good academic and social contacts made during training, there should be no fear of becoming rusty in spite of being geographically isolated. Given the right personality, enterprise and adventure, life as a GP in a remote rural area can be the most satisfying in all the important dimensions both in the short and long term—as a person, as a professional and within a family and a community

For further information	**Rural Subcommittee** BMA House Tavistock Square London WC1H 9JP Tel: 020 7388 8296 Fax: 020 7383 6911 Website: www.bma.org.uk
	Scottish Rural Subcommittee BMA House 3 Hill Place Edinburgh EH8 9EQ Tel: 0131 662 4820
	Dispensing Doctors' Association The Spinney Welford Northants NN6 7HG Website: www.dispensingdoctor.org

Royal College of General Practitioners, Rural Practice Group
Website: www.rcgp.org.uk/forums/rural/wwwboard.htm

Institute of Rural Health
Powys
Tel: 01686 650 800
Fax: 01686 650 300

Country Doctors' Association
Tel: 01858 575557
Fax: 01858 575166

WONCA Secretariat
World Organization of Family Doctors
Locked Bag 11
Collins Street East Post Office
Melbourne
Victoria 8003
Australia
Tel: +61 3 9650 0235
Fax: +61 3 9650 0236
E-mail: enquiries@wonca.org
Website: www.wonca.org/

CHAPTER 6

General (internal) medicine

Overview

General medicine covers the vast majority of hospital-based medicine. Some older physicians will tell you that everything outside the operating theatre or the laboratory is the province of the general physician. General medicine is a huge area and has been divided into increasingly smaller sub-specialties, many of which are ceding entirely from general medicine itself (e.g. paediatrics). The days of the great general physician, patrolling the wards like a Colossus, able to turn his mind to any subject and an expert in most, are coming to an end. Medicine is becoming increasingly complex and has an ever greater need for experts, although at the expense of generalists.

The 'general' aspect of internal medicine continues 'on-call' with an endless variety of different conditions making their way into hospital. Exposure to this undifferentiated on-call is essential for all doctors considering a medical (rather than surgical) career regardless of which specialty is the eventual goal. It is built into virtually every rotation and most would argue that trainees should aim to get as much 'general' experience as they can. Even when highly specialized, physicians try to maintain this generalized overview—it is considered poor form to ask in an endocrinologist simply to write up an insulin sliding scale.

All paths into general medicine start with the same two years of general training with the aim of passing both parts of the MRCP examination. After this, trainees start their specialist registrar rotation in their chosen field. Added years for experience, time abroad and research are often taken as well. Most jobs in teaching hospitals and virtually all academic posts now require a postgraduate degree, either an MD or PhD. The different pathways, therefore, vary from eight years between qualification and consultant post to 12 or more in some cases. The competitiveness of the various specialties also varies considerably; this is mentioned in the individual sections of this chapter.

General physicians are dealing with an increasingly elderly population with a consequently greater range of pathologies per patient. Therefore, as specialties are becoming ever smaller the edges and dividing lines are becoming increasingly blurred.

We have included several very small and new specialties (e.g. spinal cord injuries), not in an attempt to be desperately comprehensive but to give a feel for work in an emerging field. Every specialty listed was, at one point, a subset of a larger one.

Those branches of medicine which have their own entry exam requirements, distinct from the MRCP exam, have been listed under their own chapter headings. These include paediatrics, accident and emergency medicine and radiology.

Examinations

Medicine is unusual in not having an exit exam for specialist registrars. The MRCP exam is in the process of changing but will remain a two-part exam. Part I can be sat six months after registration and part II 18 months after registration provided enough of this has included unselected medical take. Part I consists of a notorious 60-question MCQ paper, though this should become more clinically relevant. Part II will still be a written, clinical and viva format but the written exam will be far more structured. The clinical long and short cases are being replaced by a series of objective stations (e.g. cardiovascular for 15 minutes then respiratory for 15 minutes). Precise details are available from the Royal Colleges of Physicians.

General medicine: career pathway

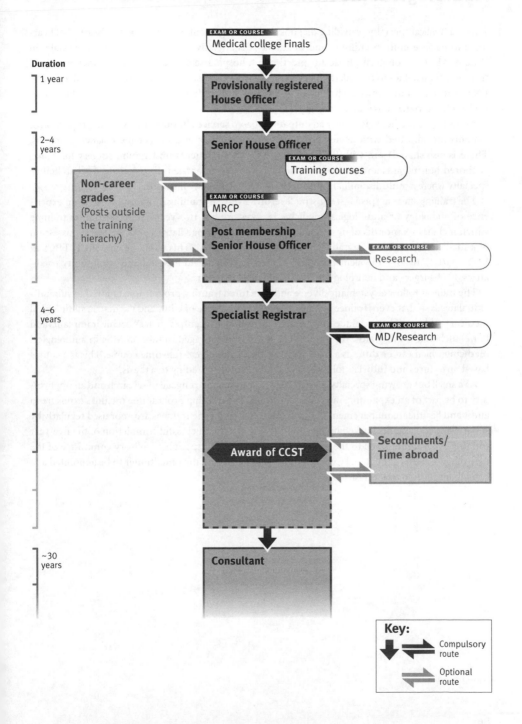

Duration

] 1 year

] 2–4 years

] 4–6 years

] ~30 years

EXAM OR COURSE
Medical college Finals

Provisionally registered House Officer

Senior House Officer

EXAM OR COURSE
Training courses

Non-career grades
(Posts outside the training hierachy)

EXAM OR COURSE
MRCP

Post membership Senior House Officer

EXAM OR COURSE
Research

Specialist Registrar

EXAM OR COURSE
MD/Research

Award of CCST

Secondments/ Time abroad

Consultant

Key:

Compulsory route

Optional route

Audiological medicine

This is a medical specialty providing diagnosis and management of patients with disorders of hearing and balance both in children and in adults. It is a relatively new but expanding specialty in Britain. Most audiological physicians practise in a hospital setting dealing with patients ranging from newborn babies to the elderly. They work closely with hospital and community paediatricians, ENT surgeons, community audiologists, geneticists, speech therapists and teachers of the deaf as well as GPs, geriatricians and neurologists.

Audiological medicine is mainly an outpatient-based service although a very small proportion of patients are admitted with acute vertigo and more complex and intractable balance problems. There is also shared care with ENT colleagues for those patients undergoing surgery for bone-anchored hearing aids and cochlear implants. It is a consultant-led diagnostic and rehabilitative specialty where a multidisciplinary approach is essential in many instances.

The training starts at specialist registrar level on a five-year training programme. No prior experience of audiology or audiological medicine is necessary but two years' postregistration training which includes six months of unselected take in medicine or paediatrics or in A&E and possession of a medical or surgical postgraduate qualification is essential. This could be an MRCP, FRCS in ENT (part 2), or an equivalent European degree. Experience in hospital and community paediatrics, ENT surgery and neurology at SHO level is advantageous.

The trainees follow a systematic diverse and structured training programme tailored to suit individual needs so that every trainee is exposed to the whole range of adult and paediatric audiological medical problems. These include those managed in specialist centres such as cochlear implants and bone-anchored hearing aids. All trainees are strongly encouraged to take an MSc in audiological medicine which can be done as a two-year part-time or one-year full-time course. This is a course based on lectures and tutorials followed by a research project leading to a thesis.

As a small but growing specialty there is tremendous scope to engage in research and an opportunity to be part of an expanding international group. The training programme includes exposure to audit and healthcare management. As with other specialties the trainees are appraised regularly by supervising consultants backed up by a monitoring system. Successful completion of the five-year training programme leads to the award of the CCST by the specialist advisory committee of the neurology section of the Royal College of Physicians enabling the practitioner to be appointed as a consultant audiological physician.

Myth	Failed ENT surgeons or laid-back physicians.
Reality	A challenging field where high-tech diagnostic methods and modern therapeutic techniques are applied with often gratifying rehabilitative results.
Personality	Tolerant, sympathetic and able to work in a team.
Best aspects	Enormous scope for research, potential to work within a small world-wide community. No on-calls and weekends free.
Worst aspects	Sometimes having to work singlehanded. Having to provide a clinical service while managing a department.
Requirements	FRCS(ENT), MRCP or equivalent

Hours

🕐 🕐 🕐 🕐 🕐   🕐 🕐 🕐 🕐 🕐

Junior   Consultant

Numbers   28 posts (5 per year)   45% are women

Competitiveness   🗡 🗡 🗡 🗡 🗡

Stress   ☹ ☹ ☹ ☹ ☹

On-calls	none	none
	Junior	Consultant

Salary

💷 £min   💷 £av   💷 £max

£50 000   £58 000   £110 000

For further information

The Secretary
British Association of Audiological Physicians
National Hospital for Neurology and Neurosurgery
Queen Square
London WC1N 3BG
Tel: 020 7837 3611
Fax: 020 7829 8775
Website: http://www.baap.org.uk

Cardiology

This is one of the most rapidly expanding fields in medicine. No other specialty within general medicine offers such a wide range of diagnostic and therapeutic procedures. It is a job for those who enjoy the intellectual rigours of internal medicine while at the same time like to do things with their hands. It encompasses an enormous array of precise diagnostic tools together with real therapeutic interventions. It is the closest to being a surgeon that a physician ever gets.

Cardiologists work in both district general hospitals and regional cardiothoracic centres. The district general hospital cardiologist usually has responsibility for a coronary care unit and takes part in the emergency take rota. The post involves treating patients with acute coronary syndromes and assessing those who will require intervention in the form of coronary angioplasty or cardiac surgery. At the regional cardiothoracic centre, the cardiologist does not usually take part in the general medical rota but works closely with the cardiac surgeons and is skilled in interventional procedures performed in the cardiac catheterization laboratory.

In the last few years the distinction between district general hospitals and regional cardiothoracic centres has become less distinct. Many district general hospitals now have cardiac catheterization suites for diagnostic work although most coronary angioplasties are still performed in the regional cardiothoracic centres. Many district general hospital cardiologists have sessions at the local regional cardiothoracic centre and perform their own angioplasties. The cardiologists at the regional cardiothoracic centres have also become more specialized as 'interventionalists' or as experts in the investigation and treatment of patients with cardiac arrhythmias. For both types of cardiologist, an interest in biotechnology and reasonable dexterity are required.

Cardiology specialist registrar training is six years long and usually begins in a district general hospital in order to acquire further experience in general medicine together with acute coronary work. This encompasses treatment of arrhythmias, the use of thrombolysis in acute myocardial infarction, the treatment of cardiogenic shock and temporary cardiac pacing. Experience in non-invasive cardiac procedures such as echocardiography, exercise stress testing and 24-hour ECG analysis is also achieved at this stage. The post then rotates to a regional cardiothoracic centre for further experience in cardiac surgery and interventional work such as coronary angioplasty. At the end of the rotation there will be an additional year in either a district general hospital or a regional cardiothoracic centre, depending on which type of job the candidate wishes to pursue in the long term. A period in research is preferable and an MD thesis will almost certainly be required if a post at a regional cardiothoracic centre is envisaged.

The workload for cardiologists is rapidly increasing with the introduction of new technologies and the greater demand from patients for access to a specialist. In district general hospitals about 30% of the daily 'take' is usually cardiology. There is a general trend towards specialization of the general take leading to a significant increase in the number of referals to cardiologists. In regional cardiothoracic centres the cardiologists are facing similar and substantial increase in referrals for intervention and arrhythmia management. Much of this work is out of hours and involves consultants.

The specialty has always been popular and competition for jobs is intense and although the workload can be very heavy in both settings, it is very rewarding with a high level of therapeutic success. A successful candidate in cardiology must be prepared to manage large numbers of patients and enjoy the satisfaction of making quick decisions, often for very sick patients in highly stressful situations. The enormous variety of the work and the satisfaction of precise diagnosis with the possibility of practical intervention are very rewarding.

Myth	Physicians who want to be surgeons
Reality	An expanding field that encompasses the best in diagnostic work together with the opportunity to perform practical and therapeutic procedures. District general hospital cardiologists can retain their interest in general medicine while regional cardiothoracic centre cardiologists may subspecialize in interventional procedures and arrhythmia work.
Personality	Generally determined individuals who enjoy acute work with precise diagnostic tools and the facility for therapeutic intervention.
Best aspects	A well-organized speciality with clear diagnostic tools and therapeutic paths. Strong emphasis on practical skills. Significant biotechnology input. Combines the best of medical diagnostics with the satisfaction of surgical therapeutics.
Worst aspects	Stressful and large workload. Emergency and out-of-hours committment can be demanding.
Requirements	MRCP

Hours

Junior   Consultant

Numbers   400 posts, rising at 35 per year   6% are women

Competitiveness

Stress

On-calls

Junior   Consultant

Salary

£55 000   £110 000   £220 000

For further information	**British Cardiac Society** 9 Fitzroy Square London W1P 5AH Tel: 020 7383 3887 Fax: 020 7388 0903 Website: www.bcs.com

Care of the elderly

Half the population in the UK survive beyond the age of 75. It is only in later life that most people now experience a breakdown in health and a restriction of daily activities. In 1900, out of a population of 38 million there were 156 000 deaths before the age of one year. In 1989, out of a population of 55 million there were 128 000 deaths before the age of 65. The very elderly (i.e. the over-85s) are still increasing rapidly in number—by over 50% during the working life of current medical students. It is this change in population patterns and disease distribution that will really test the health services of the UK in the next 20 years.

Illness in old age presents many challenges. Sometimes there are silent or atypical presentations; there is the presence of multiple aetiology and also the variability of pharmacology in old age. The situation may be yet further complicated by sociological and psychological problems.

Solution of the health problems of older people involves careful investigation and subsequent monitoring of treatment. The help of other specialties may be needed and certainly the support of workers from other disciplines is required. The geriatrician must play a central coordinating role, sometimes as advocate and protector of his or her patient. A fine balance must be drawn between a *laissez faire* or aggressive interventionist approach. Thoroughness and curiosity must be tempered by realism and compassion.

The decision to specialize in geriatric medicine is usually taken during general professional training, i.e. as an SHO. Specialist training can only be entered after passing the MRCP examination. Acquisition of the Diploma in Geriatric Medicine can be taken during SHO posts but is targeted on those doctors considering a career in general practice. However it would also show good motivation and commitment to the specialty prior to applying for a specialist registrar post on geriatric medicine.

Most specialist registrar posts provide dual training in general and geriatric medicine. If registration in both specialties is obtained, then scope for consultant posts will be wider. Most geriatricians in district general hospitals are now expected to receive emergencies of all ages when on call.

Experience in research during training is desirable but not essential. A year spent in research post-MRCP may be counted as a year's experience in geriatric medicine (but not general medicine). Full dual accreditation at specialist registrar level takes five years—two years of each specialty and one double counted for both. Specialization in geriatric medicine alone is possible (four years at specialist registrar) but consultant job opportunities may be limited in the future, probably to academic departments, in which case a higher degree is also likely to be required. Most trainees also try to gain extra expertise in specialist aspects of geriatric medicine, e.g. stroke, Parkinson's disease, diabetes or rehabilitation.

Geriatricians do not have a monopoly of elderly patients, and liaison with other departments in the management of their elderly patients is an important function. Close links have to be maintained, especially with the orthopaedic department and the department of psychiatry of old age, but advice will be sought from all hospital departments. Geriatric medicine is practised universally and is found in all district general hospitals and in all cases should have activities and responsibilities in both acute rehabilitation and continuing care. There are wide research opportunities in the major problem areas such as stroke, dementia and vascular disease.

Myth	Second-rate doctors looking after third-rate patients who are beyond hope and help.
Reality	Dealing with today's main medical challenge in the Western world (i.e. how to maintain the health, vitality and independence of an ageing population).
Personality	Innovative, empathic, resilient, tenacious, good communicator.
Best aspects	Wide range of pathology and patients with challenging problems. Close working with other specialties (e.g. old-age psychiatry and orthopaedics) and other disciplines results in a less autocratic and hierarchical specialty compared with others. Sociological, ethical and psychological elements in the work make it truly holistic but still with opportunity to have a special interest.
Worst aspects	For some, the scope of work (i.e. 'jack of all trades and master of none'). Prejudice of other specialties (i.e. ageism).
Requirements	MRCP and broad experience in medicine.

Hours

Junior   Consultant

Numbers 700 posts, more than 40 per year   14% are women
(33% of specialist registrars)

Competitiveness

Stress

On-calls

Junior   Consultant

Salary

£50 000   £62 000   £120 000

For further information	**British Geriatrics Society** 31 St John's Square London EC1M 4DN Tel: 020 7608 1369 Fax: 020 7608 1041 Website: www.bgs.org.uk

Clinical oncology

A clinical oncologist is wholly a cancer specialist, ranging from epidemiology to terminal care. The attractions of the specialty are the close patient contact, opportunities for working with other specialist teams, involvement with district medical services and openings for laboratory-based research and clinical research. Training involves reaching specified standards in all aspects of radio-therapy and oncology, which will inevitably require knowledge of physics, statistics and some mathematics. Equally important are knowledge of general and cancer medicine including chemotherapy, radiobiology and pathology. Standards are high though not daunting and the technical aspects do not at all detract from what is basically a very clinical specialty.

To become an oncologist one must first complete at least two years of general professional training at SHO level obtaining the MRCP. It will be necessary during this time to pick a rotation that includes a six-month oncology attachment. Trainees than apply for numbered specialist registrar posts in clinical oncology leading to a CCST after a five-year rotational training programme.

Once in post, the first three years are spent acquiring a full knowledge of cancer and its clinical management.

Trainees are also required to attend an approved training course in physics, medical statistics, pathology and cancer basic sciences. This may be run locally but in London the course is run by the Royal College of Radiologists. Trainees may then sit the first examination for the FRCR. Having passed this exam clinical studies begin in earnest and registrars are allowed to sit for the final examination of the Fellowship after three years in post. Formal lecture course training will continue during this time.

The final two years include secondments to other departments as well as management experience before the CCST is awarded based largely on annual assessment of your performance as a trainee. Obtaining an additional higher degree and publications from a research post are likely to give a competitive edge when applying for consultant posts.

The distinction between a clinical oncologist and medical oncologist is sometimes a little blurred at the edges. The main difference is that a medical oncologist is not trained in the use of ionizing irradiation in the treatment of cancer. At many centres, the integrated cancer service is provided by a mix of both clinical oncologists and medical oncologists. An increasing trend is for consultants to become site-specialized (e.g. in gynaecological oncology, ENT or GI tract malignancies) so that the combined team of clinical oncologists will provide a complete spectrum of clinical management skills.

In the practice of cancer medicine there is much interaction with other hospital specialist teams so that the oncologists are fully integrated members of the hospital staff and are often the main organizers of multidisciplinary treatments. Usually it is the oncologist who is responsible for out-patient follow-up which may be for many years or even for life. This leads to a close relationship with patients and their families and can be one of the most satisfying aspects of the specialty. You will also develop skills in symptom control and will be much involved in terminal care, the ultimate test of good medicine. There is not very much acute on-call commitment but as you get so close to your patients, should they become ill once more, there is an inevitable feeling of involvement which cuts across simple on-call rotas.

Myth	Machine freaks who need expensive equipment to play with because cancer is so depressing.
Reality	Hospital-based clinical medicine with surgical connections, general practice overtones and substantial research potential.
Personality	Stable, empathic and pragmatic.
Best aspects	Close patient–doctor relationship, teamwork, variety.
Worst aspects	Emotionally demanding, steadily rising workload.
Requirements	FRCR. FRCP + five years' training at an accredited centre.

Hours

Junior   Consultant

Numbers   324 posts   40% are women

Competitiveness

Stress

On-calls

Junior   Consultant

Salary

£50 000   £70 000   £120 000

For further information
Royal College of Radiologists
38 Portland Place
London W1N 4JQ
Tel: 020 7636 4432
Fax: 020 7323 3100
Website: www.rcr.ac.uk

Clinical pharmacology

Within the NHS most pure clinical pharmacologists tend to be in academic jobs (senior lecturer/ consultant physician) in medical schools, though in many district general hospitals some general physicians will have clinical pharmacology as a specialist interest. This is often put to use in drug and therapeutics, formulary and research ethics committees. Other opportunities include clinical pharmacologists in the pharmaceutical industry (at all levels of seniority up to clinical directors of major pharmaceutical companies) and serving on drug regulatory bodies such as the Committee on Safety of Medicines.

Many clinical pharmacologists have their enthusiasm sparked during their exposure to basic pharmacology in the preclinical years. Others become interested in the use of drugs when they encounter specific therapeutic problems on the wards. General medical training and the MRCP diploma are essential. Many clinical pharmacologists subsequently obtain specialty experience in a clinical subspecialty such as oncology, cardiovascular medicine or infectious disease either before, during, or after their specific training in clinical pharmacology. This may appear excessively demanding in terms of time, but consultant-level appointments are often at a relatively young age in practice.

A training programme usually involves appointment as a lecturer (with honorary status as a registrar) and it is advisable to look for a programme that is sufficiently flexible to meet your own needs. Thus, for an individual committed to a career in academic medicine it will be essential to pick a programme that provides the opportunity for substantial periods of protected time for research. The department should be one where current research activity is flourishing, that is well equipped and funded and where there is a track record of successful recent incumbents. It will be essential to join a department whose research interests fit with your own curiosity.

If you are attracted to a career in industry (which is currently keen to recruit more consultant-level clinical pharmacologists than are available on the job market) it will be an advantage to pick a programme where there is an option of spending a substantial period of time (e.g. one year) seconded to industry. This should provide experience of drug development, good clinical practice in clinical research and experience of human studies from first human dose through to clinical trials.

Training should also include appropriate clinical and teaching responsibilities and active participation in drug and therapeutics and/or formulary committees.

In summary most clinical pharmacologists are accredited both in general medicine and in clinical pharmacology by the Royal College of Physicians. However, it has to be said that this is not a subject where the number of procedures performed is of greater importance than scientific excellence (as indicated by first-author research publications) and the ability to compete successfully for outside grant support.

Myth	Modern alchemists, forever boosting shareholder profits by inventing new drugs with the letter 'z' in their name.
Reality	Very diverse career options from industry to district general, with plenty of opportunities for the non-conformist. Much scope for subspecialization in research but generalists are needed in teaching and service commitment.
Personality	Scientifically critical and professionally meticulous. Must be interested in some aspect of drugs, either how they work or how best to use them.
Best aspects	Therapeutics is such an important part of medicine and the use of medicines is such an important part of therapeutics that it's easy to stay enthusiastic and see the importance of what one is doing.
Worst aspects	At the bedside emergency no one was ever heard to cry out 'Thank goodness, here comes the clinical pharmacologist.'
Requirements	MRCP and PhD or MD

Hours

Junior ⏰⏰⏰⏰⏰   Consultant ⏰⏰⏰⏰⏰

Numbers 65 posts   5% are women

Competitiveness 🗡🗡🗡🗡🗡
depending on career goal

Stress ☹☹☹☹☹
depending on career path and personality

On-calls

Junior 📟📟📟📟📟   Consultant 📟📟📟📟📟

Salary £min £45 000   £av £70 000   £max £100 000

this is the one Caroline —
"must be interested in
SOME aspect of drugs".

Dermatology

Dermatology is a specialty that is well organized and expanding rapidly. As with most of the surgical and medical specialties, it is very poorly represented in the undergraduate curriculum at present. Most medical schools probably have no more than one month's training which prepares doctors poorly for an area of medicine that constitutes 10–15% of GP consultations.

Dermatology is largely outpatient-based with little inpatient commitment. From the service point of view it remains one of the true clinical specialties with very little requirement for high-technology support. There are, however, very good opportunities for both clinically orientated and laboratory-based research.

Dermatology has always been regarded as one of the medical specialties. Despite this, over the last 10–15 years an increasing part of the workload of a dermatologist has become surgical and it is now estimated that almost 40% of referrals to a consultant dermatologist have a surgical implication. This trend is likely to continue and the subspecialty of dermatological surgery is becoming increasingly well established. This includes complex surgical procedures and the development of cutaneous laser techniques.

Entry into the specialty is very competitive. Once in the specialty the path to accredited specialist status is fairly secure and there is plenty of work to keep the dermatologist busy. During the daytime the dermatologist works very hard but it is unusual to get called out at night or at weekends.

Training in dermatology is regulated by the specialist advisory committee of the Royal College of Physicians. Applicants for higher medical training must have completed a minimum of two years' general professional training in an approved post and obtained the MRCP qualification. One year of this must involve acute unselected medical take. Dermatology experience is not essential at this stage for enrolment into higher medical training but some exposure to dermatology is desirable and would certainly enhance the applicant's chance of getting a training-grade post. Higher medical training in dermatology takes four years in an approved training post. These training schemes are designed so that each individual will have a named trainer for each stage of higher medical training; the best schemes will have a variety of trainers throughout the course.

During the process of higher medical training the prospective dermatologist should have gained experience in the management of general dermatological problems; additional training will be expected in dermatological surgery, contact and occupational dermatitis, dermatopathology, photodermatology, paediatric dermatology and genetics, infectious diseases, genitourinary medicine, radiotherapy, dermatological oncology and the integration of dermatology in primary healthcare. It is possible, after the award of the CCST, to gain further training in a subspecialty area of dermatology to give the consultant a special expertise.

Academic dermatology is proving increasingly attractive as a career option for dermatologists and there has been an expansion in the number of academic departments. Trainees who are interested in developing an academic career are encouraged to undertake a dedicated period of research (two or three years to complete MD or PhD thesis). This can be undertaken at any time during the training programme from before entering the specialist registrar grade though the majority will enter a period of research during their training programme.

In summary, dermatology is an interesting and rewarding specialty with a great opportunity to develop subspecialty interests depending on what appeals to you during your training years.

Myth	Grease pushers who drive around in Rolls Royces. Little can be done for the patients who 'never get better but never die.'
Reality	Hard-working group of consultants with heavy clinical load. Most patients do get better in response to the correct treatment and there is considerable job satisfaction.
Personality	Straightforward realists
Best aspects	Good opportunities for clinically based and laboratory based research. Broad cross-section of patients of all ages, mostly fit and well, thus it is a predominantly outpatient specialty. Very little inpatient load.
Worst aspects	Not a mainstream acute specialty; has suffered badly in NHS reforms.
Requirements	MRCP (MD/PhD useful for jobs in major centres)

Hours

Junior ⊘⊘⊘⊘⊘   Consultant ⊘⊘⊘⊘⊘

Numbers   300 posts   ~30% are women

Competitiveness   ⚔⚔⚔⚔⚔

Stress   ☹☹☹☹☹

On-calls

Junior 📟📟📟📟📟   Consultant 📟📟📟📟📟

Salary

£50 000   £75 000   £14 000

For further information	**British Association of Dermatologists** 19 Fitzroy Square London W1P 5HQ Tel: 020 7383 0266 Fax: 020 7388 5263 Website: www.bad.org.uk
	Royal College of Physicians 11 St Andrew's Place Regent's Park London NW1 4LE Tel: 020 7935 1174 Fax: 020 7487 5218 Website: www.rcplondon.ac.uk

Endocrinology and diabetes

A career in endocrinology and diabetes can be very rewarding as it combines a high level of patient contact with long-term follow up during major life events. It is therefore inevitable that involvement with patients and their families is greater in this specialty than in many other hospital services. The discipline encourages the use of many of these skills associated with different medical specialties. These include aspects of primary and secondary care, preventative medicine and the need to preserve general medical abilities. However, this can be one of its greatest problems as the specialty is often perceived as belonging exclusively to neither the primary nor the secondary care areas, resulting in considerable administrative and funding problems in the present medical/political climate.

Although a high proportion of medical care remains consultant-led, the provision of care in both diabetes and endocrinology is team-oriented and good interpersonal skills are needed. This is because medical staff provide only a part of the overall care and work with specialist nurses, podiatrists, shoe fitters, dieticians, administrative staff and other specialist colleagues, together with all primary sector providers on a regular basis. Care is on a district basis and not only confined to acute units as in some other specialties.

Most graduates embarking on a career in diabetes and endocrinology will need to complete a two to three year rotation in general medicine and gain the MRCP before entering specialist training. This should be as broad-based as possible but time in the specialty itself, plus nephrology, neurology, cardiology and gastroenterology, would be helpful.

The next step up is into a specialist training programme which will last a variable period of time depending upon the time spent in basic research. The general aim, apart from educational considerations, is to appoint consultants nearer the age of 32 years rather than the former average of 36 years.

At least one year as a specialist registrar will be spent with a commitment to general medicine and it will be possible to opt out for periods of research. The publication of some significant research remains necessary although an MD may become optional (except for academics) and other qualifications such as an MSc may be an easier option. It will also be necessary to gain experience in subspecialist areas such as the management of diabetes in pregnancy, paediatric diabetes and endocrinology, molecular endocrinology, and the management of patients undergoing pituitary surgery.

Specialist training is still available in diabetes alone (for academics and generalists), endocrinology alone (largely for academics) and a combination of diabetes and endocrinology (mostly for generalists). Metabolic medicine has its own specialist training programme.

As in many specialties there is congestion at the stage of entering specialist registrar training while the balances required following the implementation of Calman are resolved. It may be necessary to consider time as an LAT (training locum) prior to being able to obtain a substantive post (fortunately this can be recognized retrospectively for formal training). There is also some congestion in the specialist registrar grade as there are about twice the number of candidates in training as there will be vacancies over the next three years unless there is consultant expansion.

A career in endocrinology and diabetes will suit those who wish to retain general medical skills, who appreciate a high level of patient contact and involvement and who have the personal skills of team working and patience and understanding of educational processes and counselling. Much of the work is on an outpatient basis and this emphasizes the need for considerable administrative skills and a high level of ability to tolerate more clinics than in other disciplines.

Myth	Laid-back physicians who seem to invent insulin doses with ease.
Reality	Good communication skills; listening to patients; attention to detail. Although most skills are verbal there is a high scientific basis to the specialty.
Personality	Apparently calm, but often pedantic and with serious attention to detail.
Best aspects	Technical specialty but requiring verbal as well as practical skills. Good training programmes. Research involves high scientific content.
Worst aspects	Personally very demanding because of emotional nature of many patient problems and high consultant involvement in providing immediate clinical care. This can, of course, be one of the most rewarding aspects of this specialty.
Requirements	MRCP (MD for most jobs)

Hours

Junior   Consultant

Numbers   380 posts   8% are women

Competitiveness

Stress

On-calls

Junior   Consultant

Salary

£50 000   £65 000   £80 000

For further information	**Royal College of Physicians** 11 St Andrew's Place Regent's Park London NW1 4LE Tel: 020 7935 1174 Fax: 020 7487 5218 Website: www.rcplondon.ac.uk

Gastroenterology

The specialty of gastroenterology has expanded tremendously since the advent of fibre-optic endoscopy 30 years ago, which has allowed visual examination of the gastrointestinal (GI) tract. GI diseases are very common; one in three adults suffer from indigestion in any month and GI diseases cause one in six of all hospital admissions and one in 10 of deaths in the UK. Cancer of the large bowel is the second commonest cancer in the UK.

Gastroenterology is a branch of internal medicine and gastroenterologists are physicians who investigate and treat patients with GI disorders, including diseases of the liver, pancreas and biliary tree. Gastroenterologists work closely with gastrointestinal surgeons, radiologists and pathologists. Because of endoscopy and other investigative techniques, gastroenterologists need to have considerable technical expertise and manual dexterity. Medical gastroenterologists will treat many disorders, e.g. oesophageal strictures or common duct gall stones, by endoscopic therapeutic techniques which, before the advent of endoscopy, would have been treated surgically.

The gastroenterologist needs to be a physician who is caring and understanding of his (or her) patients' needs and considers the whole patient, but at the same time he (or she) needs a surgical temperament because he (or she) will perform diagnostic and therapeutic procedures on patients which can occasionally go wrong. At present, most gastroenterologists in hospitals in the UK take part in the acute general medical on-take rota and therefore need a good grounding in general internal medicine. A few gastroenterologists practice entirely in liver diseases. These hepatologists tend to work in major teaching centres where liver transplantation is performed. A tiny minority of gastroenterologists will deal with children and will need a good training in paediatric medicine.

The career path for a gastroenterologist is the standard pathway for internal medicine. Although not a requirement of CCST, most gastroenterologists, and especially those who aspire to a consultant post in a teaching hospital or on an academic unit, will need to do a period of research in gastroenterology leading to a higher degree (MD or PhD). This can be done before specialist registrar training or during time taken out of the registrar training programme. Up to 12 months for research may be taken out of the five-year period of specialist registrar training without delaying the CCST date.

Having a 'procedure' leads to good opportunities for private practice but also ensures that the NHS practice remains very busy. This is with both emergency needs as well as the planned workload.

Myth	Only interested in technical procedures such as endoscopy; frustrated surgeons.
Reality	An enjoyable specialty which has the benefit of practising medicine combined with the enjoyment of using sophisticated investigative and therapeutic techniques which require considerable manual skills.
Personality	Thoughtful, practical, able to communicate with patients and colleagues (especially surgeons).
Best aspects	Technical aspects (e.g. endoscopy); application of science to the disease.
Worst aspects	Acute medicine on-call during training.
Requirements	MRCP (MD/PhD for jobs in major centres)

Hours

Junior   Consultant

Numbers   450 posts   10% are women

Competitiveness

Stress

On-calls

Junior   Consultant

Salary

£min   £av   £max

£50 000   £75 000   £150 000

For further information	**British Society of Gastroenterology** 3 St Andrew's Place Regents Park London NW1 4LB Tel: 020 7935 2815 Fax: 020 7487 3734 Website: www.bsg.org.uk	**Royal College of Physicians** 11 St Andrew's Place Regent's Park London NW1 4LE Tel: 020 7935 1174 Fax: 020 7487 5218 Website: www.rcplondon.ac.uk

Genitourinary medicine (sexual health medicine)

A national network of clinics for the diagnosis and treatment of sexually transmitted infections (STIs) was set up following the report of a Royal Commission on venereal diseases in 1916. The name of the specialty evolved from 'venereology' to the rather obscure title of 'genitourinary medicine' and there are currently moves to change it to sexual health medicine.

As the change in title implies, there has been a shift in emphasis from concentrating on disease to looking towards sexual health promotion as an integral part of the role of this specialty. The epidemiology of sexually transmitted infections (STIs) has also shifted from readily treatable bacterial infections such as gonorrhoea to less easily managed viral infections including human papilloma virus, herpes simplex virus and the human immunodeficiency virus (HIV). The emergence of HIV led to a renaissance in interest in STIs and a large influx of money to develop services, allowing the expansion and modernization of what was previously perceived to be a 'Cinderella' specialty.

The sexual health specialist needs a firm grounding in general medicine, gynaecology (including family planning), dermatology and HIV medicine; an interest in psychosexual medicine is also useful. Open-mindedness and a non-judgmental attitude are essential. On the whole, we look after a relatively young and fit group of patients with readily treatable conditions.

There is still great scope for research into STIs, particularly into factors leading to spread of infections within communities and subsections of communities. The academic profile of the specialty has been enhanced by the creation of a number of specific Chairs in genitourinary medicine; a diploma course in the specialty is run in Liverpool and London.

A six-month stint as a Senior House Officer is recommended to ensure that you and the specialty are compatible. The specialty may be accessed via MRCP, or MRCOG, the latter being more time consuming due to the requirement to do an additional 12 months general medicine. Those arriving via the medical route would be expected to gain some O&G experience. Higher specialist training, at SpR level, lasts four years with the possibility of additional research.

The first two years are used to develop a sound grounding in the epidemiology, diagnosis, clinical management and complications of common genital complaints. Competence in the management of HIV, dealing with contraceptive advice and the development of counselling and partner notification skills are also gained. The final two years are spent developing specialist interests (e.g. colposcopy, vulval clinics etc.). The inpatient management of HIV is now an integral part of the training grade. That said, most jobs involve predominantly outpatient work with a limited inpatient commitment and that rare commodity in medicine—social working hours.

Myth	An obscure branch of medicine, best kept at arm's length, in which doctor and patient are hard to tell apart.
Reality	An increasingly dynamic and competitive field which rapidly developed with the advent of HIV infection in the early 1980s.
Personality	Diverse, but generally trendier than your average physician.
Best aspects	Generally, a healthy patient group with curable conditions; social working hours. Ample opportunities for special interests.
Worst aspects	Narrow spectrum of conditions.
Requirements	MRCOG/MRCP

Hours

🕐 🕐 🕐 🕐 🕐   🕐 🕐 🕐 🕐 🕐

Junior   Consultant

Numbers   220 posts   19% are women

Competitiveness

🗡 🗡 🗡 🗡 🗡

Stress

☹ ☹ ☹ ☹ ☹

On-calls

📟 📟 📟 📟 📟   📟 📟 📟 📟 📟

Junior   Consultant

Salary

£min   £av   £max

£50 000   £62 000   £75 000

For further information

Medical Society for the Study of Venereal Diseases
Royal Society of Medicine
1 Wimpole Street
London W1M 8AE
Tel: 020 7290 2900
Fax: 020 7290 2989
Website: www.mssvd.org.uk

Royal College of Physicians
11 St Andrew's Place
Regent's Park
London NW1 4LE
Tel: 020 7935 1174
Fax: 020 7487 5218
Website: www.rcplondon.ac.uk

Infectious diseases and tropical medicine

This is a 'Cinderella' specialty with the same number of trainees nationwide in the UK as in a single major city in the USA. Historically, infectious diseases medicine has a very humble ancestry in fever hospitals, which were quite inferior academically and distinct geographically from teaching hospitals. Another blight to the study of infectious diseases medicine was the legacy of high-profile UK microbiologists like Fleming who bequeathed the idea that all physicians needed was antibiotic advice. Infections as clinical problems were dead and buried. Tropical medicine has roots in the colonial medical service and is now associated with travel medicine, geographical medicine, imported infections, emergency medicine, overseas aid and development, or parasitic disease.

However, as a modern specialty, infectious diseases and tropical medicine (ITDM) is second to none for variety and job satisfaction. The ITDM consultant should have a thorough experience of acute medical need. They will have seen it all and done it all, preferably by prolonging their specializing, so the path is long. A knowledge of microbiology and virology, immunology, parasitology and therapeutics is compulsory. Dermatology and genitourinary medicine should also be studied. Research is also necessary, typically in immunology or microbiology, and a PhD or MD will be expected. This is a hands-on specialty with heavy on-call commitments until retirement.

A two-year general medical SHO rotation ending in the MRCP is the starting point for the specialty. In the UK, no two consultants are identical in their training or strengths. The new specialist registrar grade will homogenize this somewhat with a typical five-year programme in ITDM combining general internal medicine with an interest in respiratory or gastrointestinal medicine (one year), microbiology/virology (one year), HIV/genitourinary medicine (one year) and ITDM (two years). This is still too brief for the job requirements, so extra years of research (two to three years, possibly in the tropics) and more years of clinical work (e.g. in the tropics or USA) will undoubtedly be added. Expect to be older, wiser and poorer than your colleagues but richer in experience. You can claim no procedure (scope or catheterization) as a unique part of your job, so your private practice earnings will be comparatively low: make this into a virtue.

It is misconception about tropical medicine that you can spend your career working six months in the UK and six months abroad. No NHS hospital will tolerate this. Wanderlust is generally satisfied by research projects in the field. This is often undertaken precariously by your juniors or other collaborators, or by 'study leave' if you can wangle it. For this reason try to work abroad as often and whenever you can. Tropical centres are few and far between and as a tropical doctor you will be teaching or serving on committees, building links with overseas institutions, trying to get research grants to study tropical diseases, seeing patients with imported diseases and possibly travelling abroad to do a drug trial, control an epidemic, study pathophysiology or collect bugs.

Some infectious disease physicians exclusively look after immunocompromised patients (e.g. those with HIV infection or leukaemia, or those taking steroids); others cater for conditions such as chickenpox, diarrhoea, etc. Some mix laboratory research (typically with molecular biology, parasitology and immunology) and clinical work. ITDM often takes the best parts of acute general medicine, like the young previously fit patients with life-threatening infections such as meningitis, pneumonia and septicaemia.

Myth	Glamorous international experts who spend months abroad each year sorting out Ebola outbreaks then return to the NHS when they feel like it.
Reality	A small 'Cinderella' speciality with very long training, highly competitive, and with no certainty of a job at the end of it all. Once a consultant, job satisfaction is superb.
Personality	Must love hands-on clinical work and also like laboratory work.
Best aspects	The diagnostic challenge, acutely ill patients who are cured if you are correct. Lots of teaching, overseas contacts, and overlaps with other specialities.
Worst aspects	Very long training with no clear role model to follow at first. Colleagues jealous of your interesting patients and almost no private practice prospects.
Requirements	MRCP and PhD or MD also DTM&H or MSc in microbiology advisable.

Hours

Junior   Consultant

Numbers   60 posts, 2 or 3 per year   almost no women

Competitiveness

Stress

On-calls

Junior   Consultant

Salary   £min   £av   £max

£50 000   £55 000   £65 000

For further information	**Royal College of Physicians** 11 St Andrew's Place Regent's Park London NW1 4LE Tel: 020 7935 1174 Fax: 020 7487 5218 Website: http://www.rcplondon.ac.uk

Medical oncology

There have only been doctors specializing in the drug treatment of cancer since the 1960s. Until the past few years almost all medical oncologists were based in academic departments funded by the major cancer charities, the Cancer Research Campaign or the Imperial Cancer Research Fund. Since the 1980s most radiotherapy departments have appointed at least one medical oncologist. The 1990s saw a rapid expansion in the number of medical oncologists as various trials have demonstrated the survival benefit of chemotherapy for patients with common cancers such as breast and colon cancers. This has resulted in major district general hospitals appointing a medical oncologist so that they can safely offer patients chemotherapy on site, and be classified as a cancer unit. A large number of consultant posts remain associated with academic departments as either NHS appointments or university appointments for those wishing to become a professor eventually.

There have been more advances in the care of patients with cancer over the past 30 years than in any other field of medicine. Progress is likely to be even more rapid in the future. Medical oncologists must therefore be able to keep up with the latest advances and be capable of changing the way they manage patients. This requires that medical oncologists are trained both to participate in trials of new therapies and to analyse critically other people's research. It is likely that the majority of medical oncologists will maintain a research commitment.

Medical oncologists have historically differed from radiotherapists (who are now called clinical oncologists and belong to the Royal College of Radiology) in being more academic. This has arisen because the clinical oncologists have had to supervise radiotherapy and chemotherapy for so many patients, often in different hospitals, that they had no time to enter patients into clinical trials. Medical oncologists are only involved in the drug treatment of cancer and are expected to specialize in certain types of cancer. They require excellent communication skills and the ability to make often difficult decisions as to the best way to manage a particular patient.

Applicants for the specialist registrar grade in medical oncology must have completed a minimum of two years at SHO level with at least one year of this period involving acute unselected medical intake. A period as an SHO in medical oncology is desirable. After attainment of the MRCP it is necessary to apply for an approved and numbered higher specialist training post. Attendance at an oncology lecture course is recommended during this period. Trainees manage many patients on the wards and have regular clinics, but major decisions are made with close supervision.

The higher training phase consists of at least two years' in-depth specialist training including involvement in studies of new therapies and the delivery of more complex and intensive chemotherapy regimens. Time is spent with different site specialists. It is expected that most medical oncologists will spend an additional two to three years in a research project leading to a higher degree. The senior trainee will be expected to decide on treatment options which extend from deciding whether chemotherapy is appropriate to the optimal chemotherapy regimen. There is regular assessment by consultants but no exit examination. This allows some trainees to devote their time to acquiring a highly specialized interest that can be pursued further once they become a consultant.

Myth	Depressives who go round poisoning patients.
Reality	A specialty where there are exciting advances in new therapies and in ways to overcome the toxicity of the therapy.
Personality	Communication skills essential but could be a research boffin.
Best aspects	So much one can do for patients from controlling symptoms such as pain, through temporary tumour shrinkage, to curing widespread disease.
Worst aspects	Emotionally demanding as patients can be very ill and many die.
Requirements	MRCP and PhD or MD

Hours

🕐 🕐 🕐 🕐 🕐   🕐 🕐 🕐 🕐 🕐

Junior   Consultant

Numbers   112 posts (3–25 per year)   13% are women

Competitiveness

Stress   ☹ ☹ ☹ ☹ ☹

On-calls

Junior   Consultant

Salary

£50 000   £70 000   £120 000

For further information	**Royal College of Physicians** 11 St Andrew's Place Regent's Park London NW1 4LE Tel: 020 7935 1174 Fax: 020 7487 5218 Website: www.rcplondon.ac.uk

Nuclear medicine

'It must be very claustrophobic in those submarines', said a lady at a dinner party to my colleague recently—admitting you are a nuclear physician is better than saying you're the man who invented traffic cones at stopping dinner party conversation. Why would anybody allow themselves to be tortured in this way: why not admit to being a dog catcher or a radiologist?! Well, nuclear medicine has little to do with nuclear submarines, nuclear bombs or splitting the atom. It has a lots to do with following the physiological processes in the body using radioactive tracers. These use minute amounts ($<10^9$ g) of a pharmaceutical linked to a radioisotope to follow a physiological or pathological process in the patient (such as the blood supply to cardiac muscle or the the flow of tears through a tear duct). It is possible to follow the response of brain dopamine receptors in patients treated for Parkinson's diseases and monitor the effect of chemotherapy on a patient's breast cancer. As many nuclear medicine tests are considered 'routine', the need for extended working and 'on-call' commitment increases.

If you are the kind of person who still looks at *New Scientist* and remembers the time when science was exciting and learning was about exploration of the world, not learning the Latin names for various nerves and muscles, nuclear medicine is for you. Flexible training and working is not uncommon and the proportion of female winners of merit awards in nuclear medicine is among the highest in medicine, showing that women are not just there to 'make up the numbers' but are an important and integral part of the specialty.

Exciting new developments have meant that nuclear medicine is not just about imaging patients: increasingly nuclear physicians are called upon to treat patients, particularly those with cancer in whom other treatment has failed. This has led to an increase in clinic and ward work. This is very satisfying but there are drawbacks as it increases workload and stress without normally resulting in an increase in resources.

Entry into nuclear medicine full time is normally after completion of general professional training and gaining MRCP or MRCS. Nuclear medicine can be a stand-alone subject (needing four years of higher professional training for a nuclear physician). It can be part of radiology training with a one- or two-year course. The longer the training the more that you can do clinically and the more time is devoted to practice of nuclear medicine. Therapy is normally only given by nuclear physicians. A government committee (ARSAC) regulates nuclear medicine and grants licences for relevant tests appropriate to training. For example, a nuclear radiologist with one year's training can perform simple diagnostic tests, one with two years' training can perform almost all diagnostic tests, whilst one with four years' training can do all diagnostic and therapeutic procedures he or she is trained in. Though it is not essential, it is recommended that all nuclear physicians in training and some nuclear radiologists (with two years' training) take and pass an MSc in nuclear medicine and this has been reformulated in modular form to assist in distance learning.

Research remains an essential area of nuclear medicine and is encouraged not just in junior staff trying to get a job—even senior consultants will be working on their favourite projects. The number of posts has been growing slowly over the past four years as it is recognized that it is often more cost-effective to have larger departments run by full-time enthusiasts than looked after by a radiologist with other interest. Nuclear medicine physician posts are no longer restricted to university hospitals.

Myth	Often seen as a mixture of Merlin and Einstein, who dresses badly, has untidy hair and speaks mumbo-jumbo.
Reality	Scientific discipline; *in vivo* physiologists; expanding field of new techniques; no two are days the same. Dress and hair: no comment.
Personality	Able to communicate well with your clinical colleagues to whom you provide a service, but tough enough to gain the resources you need.
Best aspects	Scientific discipline, good for those who do not wish to follow the crowd, who ask questions; varied; part-time work is no problem.
Worst aspects	Can be lonely if working on your own. Poor resources.
Requirements	CCST in nuclear medicine; MSc in nuclear medicine. MRCP or FRCR advisable.

Hours

Junior   Consultant

Numbers   40 posts (1 or 2 per year)   25% are women

Competitiveness

Stress

On-calls

Junior   Consultant

Salary

£50 000   £70 000   £90 000

For further information
British Nuclear Medicine Society
1 Wimpole Street
London W1G 0AE
Tel: 020 8291 7800
Fax: 020 8699 2227
Website: bnms.org.uk

Neurology

Neurological practice has changed enormously in the last few years. The main element of this change is due to changes in patterns of referral: common neurological diseases such as migraine and epilepsy, once dealt with largely by general physicians, are increasingly regarded as neurology core business and are sent to neurologists. The main consequence of this is that life in neurology is dominated by the fact that there is more neurology about than a small specialty can cope with. Expansion of posts has fought a rearguard action against this problem, rather than defeating it, and this is likely to continue. So, if you become a neurologist, expect pressure in your daily clinical work. Increasingly, the on-call neurology team is expected to deal with emergencies, so there is more urgent and emergency work than there once was.

Luckily, change has brought about good news too. Much of that is due to a recent explosion in new therapies for neurological disease. This has meant that neurologists spend less time diagnosing rare and untreatable conditions, and more time taking crucial patient management decisions. Diagnostic advances have changed neurological practice dramatically: structural and functional imaging techniques allow us to see inside the central nervous system in ways not dreamed of 20 years ago and advances in clinical neurophysiology and molecular biology have revolutionized diagnosis in other ways. Having said all that, clinical skills remain more important than in most specialties. For example, the prime diagnostic criteria remain clinical in disorders such as epilepsy and migraine.

A relatively high proportion of neurologists work in regional centres, usually along with neurosurgeons, neuroradiologists and clinical neurophysiologists. Many working in such centres have subspecialized into areas such as epilepsy, movement disorders (e.g. Parkinson's disease) and cerebrovascular medicine.

Getting into neurology is competitive: most successful candidates for specialist registrar posts will already have some neurology experience and may already have spent a period in research. The training programme lasts five years. Competition for consultant posts is also likely to be stiff for the foreseeable future. Neurology provides a good opportunity for private practice and for medicolegal work, and the latter is often interesting and challenging.

You will not get an easy life in neurology, but you will get an interesting one. If you don't mind hard work, like patient contact and like diagnostic detective work, then neurology may be for you.

Myth	Dry, dusty eccentrics who like to categorize rare untreatable syndromes.
Reality	High-tech approaches to diagnosis and a recent explosion in therapeutic options have propelled neurology into the 21st century.
Personality	All sorts, but with a bias toward the academically inclined.
Best aspects	Patient contact skills still highly important. Lots of high-tech toys for those inclined towards physics; increasing amounts of molecular biology and genetics for the test-tube fans.
Worst aspects	There is high-pressure demand for neurology so many posts are very busy requiring a 'sausage factory' approach to outpatient work.
Requirements	MRCP (MD/PhD for most jobs)

Hours

Junior   Consultant

Numbers 310 posts (10–15 per year) 12% are women

Competitiveness

Stress

On-calls

(more in district general hospitals)

Junior   Consultant

Salary

£50 000   £75 000   £100 000

For further information	**Association of British Neurologists** Ormond House 4th Floor 27 Boswell Street London WC1N 3JZ Tel: 020 7405 4060 Fax: 020 7405 4070 E-mail: abn@abnoffice.demon.co.uk

Occupational medicine

Occupational medicine is a diverse and growing clinical speciality. The prime concern of the specialist occupational physician is to look after the health of the working population, in terms of both assessing the impact of work on health and dealing with the effects of ill health on an individual's ability to work. To achieve this means achieving a degree of competence in a number of areas, as well as working with a wide variety of other Health and Safety Executive (HSE) professionals and people at all levels in the chosen area of business.

In the UK, the NHS has no responsibility for providing occupational health services to the general population, nor is there a general statutory requirement—as there is in some countries—for all employers to make occupational health available to all workers. Recently, however, with the changing nature of industry and the decline in the UK manufacturing base, the trend appears to be away from the resulting piecemeal in-house services towards independent providers delivering contract services to many organizations on a regional or even a national basis, and providing an essential resource to small and medium enterprises—a particular concern of the Government at present.

The curriculum for specialist training is a broad one. Topics for study include a thorough grounding in the health hazards of the work environment (physical, chemical, biological, ergonomic and psychosocial) as well as the principles of measurement, risk evaluation, control and monitoring, the assessment of disability and fitness for work, principles of epidemiology and statistics, occupational health law and ethics, environmental medicine, health promotion, principles of management and the organization and structure of industry. The list is substantial and extends beyond the boundaries of most other areas of medical training.

Because of the nature of the speciality, getting into training may present some challenges. Following registration, a period of general professional training, as an SHO in a relevant hospital discipline or on a GP vocational training rotation is mandatory, and a higher qualification (MRCGP or MRCP) is helpful in securing a training post. Beyond this point, there are both NHS and non-NHS training posts available: the latter have to be approved by the Specialist Advisory Committee of the JCHMT. This process, and the costs of training within an approved post in a commercial environment, may place a significant burden on an employer and the number of jobs available is limited.

Once you have qualified there is a wide variety of career opportunities. There are certainly opportunities for those of an entrepreneurial nature, though in a robust and competitive business environment, the occupational health physician may face repeated demands to show the cost–benefit of the service. He or she needs to enjoy producing practical solutions to meet the needs of businesses, without compromising ethical standards and recognizing the conflict that may arise.

Some larger organizations have substantial in-house services where the occupational physician may have the responsibility for organizing and managing the department. Occupational health specialists are increasingly being recruited to public services such as the police and fire services and educational establishments. The NHS is now establishing many new consultant and specialist training jobs, and some departments are selling services on a commercial basis to local companies and organizations. The armed services recognize occupational medicine as a speciality and have a number of training posts, which may be linked to related areas such as aviation medicine. Research and teaching posts are available in a number of academic departments. The HSE employs occupational medicine specialists to advise their own inspectorates as well as giving guidance to businesses, employees and unions.

Myth	Doctors whose key role is to perform endless routine screening medicals, in between playing golf with the MD.
Reality	A wide range of jobs that are as varied as the organizations they serve. A mix of: understanding the risks arising from work; health promotion; environmental medicine; managerial aspects; research; and teaching; all supported by a firm clinical foundation.
Personality	Good interpersonal skills; can communicate across all levels; persuasive; able to produce innovative and practical solutions; wants to survive and thrive in a commercial environment.
Best aspects	Variety; making a real difference to peoples' working lives; many challenges; possibility of travel; can develop own areas of special interest and expertise.
Worst aspects	Regularly having to face demands to demonstrate the value of occupational health services; turbulence and reorganization in industry; possibly a higher degree of job uncertainty than in the NHS; may be limited career development unless one is prepared to move between organizations
Requirements	MFOM, other clinical qualifications an advantage
Hours	🕐 🕐 🕐 🕐 🕐
Numbers	1000 posts in full/part-time work
Competitiveness	🗡 🗡 🗡 🗡 🗡
Stress	☹ ☹ ☹ ☹ ☹
On-calls	📟 📟 📟 📟 📟
Salary	£min £av £max
	£45 000 £65 000 £120 000
For further information	**Faculty of Occupational Medicine of the Royal College of Physicians** 6 St Andrews Place Regents Park London NW1 4LB Tel: 020 7317 5890 Fax: 020 7317 5899 Website: http://www.facoccmed.ac.uk/	**The Society of Occupational Medicine** *same address as left* Tel: 020 7486 2641 Fax: 020 7486 0028 Website: www.som.org.uk

Ophthalmology

Ophthalmology combines aspects of medicine and surgery in a way that no other medical specialty does, adding elements of physics and perceptual psychology in good measure. It is often represented rather thinly in the busy undergraduate timetable, so that a fleeting contact with the subject at medical school, together with the dark mysteries of optics and the strange virtual world of the indirect ophthalmoscope may discourage the newly qualified doctor from considering ophthalmology as an option when wondering what to do with his future. This would be a great mistake, as it is a hugely rewarding profession, having quality, not quantity, as its currency and providing opportunities for the expression of intellectual and manual skills in equal measure.

Ophthalmological diagnosis employs a very diverse range of techniques: eliciting and interpreting clinical signs by observation and the performance of unique special tests, including optical (refraction), neurophthalmological (perimetry and eye movement assessment), physical (tonometry) and perceptual methods which have no parallel in any other field. Moreover, the great majority of investigations can be carried out by the ophthalmologist in the consulting room with small and elegant instruments, and accurate diagnosis can almost always be made by clinical means at the time of presentation.

This very satisfactory situation extends to treatment, which can similarly be managed on a humane scale between ophthalmologist and patient without the need for big noisy machines, messy tubes, painful experiences or intensive care. Patient and doctor both derive very great satisfaction from the restoration of lost sight.

The precise and well-made instruments used in eye surgery and the image of the surgical field in the operating microscope sometimes seem to recall jewellery or art more than surgery. While cataract surgery must be one of the most rewarding operations in any surgical field, restoring clearer sight than any patients can believe possible, other kinds of operation undertaken in the eye theatre include concepts more arcane than simply replacing an opaque lens in the eye with a clear one while a pianist plays Schubert on the CD. In retinal surgery, for example, the retina itself must not be touched or directly instrumented; tissues can be divided or coagulated remotely and non-mechanically using a laser beam of great brightness and beauty. Also, in surgery to correct strabismus, the movement of the eyes may be adjusted postoperatively when the patient has awakened, and so can tell the surgeon exactly how much to adjust the muscles in order to join diplopia (double vision) to binocular single visions.

Ophthalmology embraces not only its own peculiar and unique range of disorders, but extends to involve most other field of medicine and surgery—not only diabetes and hypertension, but also neurology, endocrine disease, rheumatology, oncology, paediatrics—and even venereology, may express themselves as eye diseases. The field is therefore a very broad one, and far from confining himself (or herself) to a small organ of no more than a cubic inch in size, the good ophthalmologist needs to be real physician who understands his/her patient as a whole.

Training consists of at least three years at SHO level completing the three parts of the MRCOphth exam then optional research and four and a half years as an specialist registrar with the FRCOphth as the exit exam. The reward will be a practice which is never repetitive, but always challenging and stimulating, calling upon all the intellectual and practical talents the ophthalmologist has. They will have very many appreciative patients and will seldom be called from their bed in the small hours of the night.

Myth	Ophthalmology is cataract surgery with obscure and difficult physics and endless elderly patients.
Reality	Very diverse—challenging diagnosis, marvellous instrumentation, highly rewarding surgery and very happy patients.
Personality	More varied than the average surgeon; keen on detail.
Best aspects	Combination of science, medicine and surgery into a potentially highly creative package. Civilized out-of-hours commitment.
Worst aspects	Very busy clinics. Very demanding surgery in which failure or complication is always very close and has potentially catastrophic consequences.
Requirements	FRCOphth. Stereoscopic vision.

Hours

Junior   Consultant

Numbers 605 posts   12% are women

Competitiveness

Stress

On-calls

Junior   Consultant

Salary

£50 000   £90 000   £500 000

For further information

Royal College of Ophthalmologists
17 Cornwall Terrace
London NW1 4QW
Tel: 020 7935 0702
Fax: 020 7935 9838
Website: www.rcophth.ac.uk

Palliative medicine

A palliative physician provides the medical component of palliative care. She, or less often, he, will work alongside the other professionals in the team caring for patients and their families. Palliative medicine deals with patients whose diseases are incurable and where the purpose of treatment is to control symptoms and relieve distress. It is an intensely clinical specialty, which has grown more rapidly than any other in the last decade. It was recognized as a specialty by the Royal Colleges of Physicians (RCP) in 1987.

Palliative care has evolved from the modern hospice movement, which dates from the opening of St Christopher's Hospice, Sydenham, London, by Dame Cicely Saunders in 1967. However, there have been hospices since mediaeval times, and perhaps palliative care is a rediscovery and reaffirmation of old values rather than a completely new discipline. Until the last 25 years it was more likely to be called terminal care or care of the dying, and could only be practised outside the NHS in the charitable sector.

To train in palliative medicine, it is necessary as an SHO to complete two years' General Professional Training (GPT). This can be more broadly based than other medical specialties. However, it must include at least 18 months' experience in the admission and early follow-up of acute emergencies, six months of which must be 'acute, unselected, medical take'. Some time spent as a general practice vocational trainee is allowable. One of the following postgraduate diplomas must be obtained: MRCP, MRCGP, FRCA or FRCR (in clinical oncology).

Entry to the specialist registrar grade is currently highly competitive. Nearly 80% of specialist registrars are female and 30% train flexibly. The length of Higher Specialist Training (HST) is four years full-time, although this is longer proportionately for flexible trainees. All deaneries have rotational schemes which include hospice, hospital and community experience. Research is encouraged and some rotations have opportunities to pursue full-time research projects. Only one year of research can count towards HST.

Traditionally, palliative medicine is concerned predominantly with advanced cancer and motor neuron disease; however, there is also interest and pressure to include many other progressive incurable illnesses such as end-stage heart and respiratory failure and various symptom-control problems including chronic pain.

Consultant posts have been increasing rapidly recently (300% over the last five years). At the time of writing there is a considerable shortage of applicants for consultant posts. Therefore once a CCST is obtained, there is little difficulty in gaining a consultant appointment. However, the new appointee may find herself in a new post without adequate support yet in place. She may be required to design and implement the new service as well as making the case for other consultant or junior colleagues.

The Calman Report has recognized palliative medicine as an essential component of the team in all three cancer-care locations: centre, unit, and community. This has brought the palliative physician into the hospitals from the hospices and community.

The hospice movement generally, and palliative medicine in particular, are products of the British healthcare system. There has been great interest abroad and most countries are now starting to build their own palliative care structures. There is heavy demand for speakers and teachers to travel abroad. For those who enjoy exchanging ideas with foreign colleagues there are unrivalled opportunities for travel, although there is rarely any financial reward.

Myth	Do-gooding pious hand-holders.
Reality	Demanding medically and psychologically. One of the most intensely clinical of all specialties. Empathy but also toughness are essential. Only the well balanced will survive. Owes more to true team work than most disciplines.
Personality	Caring, compassionate and able to handle raw emotions.
Best aspects	Genuine gratitude from patients and relatives. The opportunity to help in people's life crises. Involvement in the new specialty. Humbling and loyal voluntary support. The learning opportunities of team work, especially from nursing colleagues. Being welcome both in hospital and at home.
Worst aspects	Psychological battle fatigue. The obduracy of those that have been 'called'. Nursing philosophy that views palliative medicine as only opioid prescription. The fear that delaying until tomorrow may be too late.
Requirements	MRCP, MRCGP, FRCA, or FRCR

Hours

Junior ⏰⏰⏰🕐🕐   Consultant ⏰⏰⏰🕐🕐

Numbers 250 posts (40 per year)   >50% are women

Competitiveness 🗡🗡🗡🗡🗡
to enter specialist registrar grade

Stress ☹☹☹☹☹

On-calls

Junior 📟📟📟📟📟   Consultant 📟📟📟📟📟

Salary £min £av £max
£50 000   £60 000   £80 000

For further information	**The Association for Palliative Medicine of Great Britain and Ireland** 11 Westwood Road Southampton SO17 1DL Tel: 01703 672888 E-mail: apmsecretariat@claranet.co.uk Website: www.palliative-medicine.org

Renal medicine

This is a small specialty but is growing as a result of a continued increase in the numbers of patients being kept alive on dialysis treatment, many of whom are not candidates for transplantation as a result of age or co-existing disease. Most large district hospitals now have a dialysis unit; transplantation is performed only in larger centres.

Nephrologists can get by without detailed understanding of renal physiology but require a good working knowledge of immunology (for management of systemic vasculitis, glomerulonephritis and transplantation) and of the management of infections and of hypertension. Now that elderly patients are not automatically refused treatment, the majority of patients are elderly. Around 40% of all consultant nephrologists in the UK do general medical 'takes', the remainder concentrating solely on patients with renal disease. All require good grounding in general medicine, as nephrologists often have to manage general medical problems occurring in patients with chronic renal disease.

Nephrologists work in close collaboration with surgeons (who construct arteriovenous fistulae, insert peritoneal dialysis catheters and perform kidney transplants), urologists (caring for patients with abnormal urinary tracts resulting in renal damage from obstruction or infection), dialysis nurses and technicians, and many other specialities, given that acute renal failure can complicate a wide range of conditions. In particular, good working relationships are needed with transplant surgeons, who (rightly) don't like being treated as technicians. In some hospitals, nephrologists have a major role in the provision of renal support for patients with multi-organ failure on the intensive care unit but in others this role is largely taken by intensivists/anaesthetists.

Nephrology is very much a 'hands-on' specialty, including insertion of many types of dialysis catheter and ultrasound-guided percutaneous renal biopsy. Patients with end-stage renal failure are stuck with their nephrologist for life. They often have long medical histories, and can appear demanding, particularly when faced with a junior doctor who knows much less about their condition than they do! Many present to the renal unit with medical problems unrelated to their renal disease. Successful care of these patients requires compassion and long-term commitment. Continuity of care, over many years, of a small number of complicated patients brings enormous rewards.

Research training is not required but many trainees take time out, usually to do laboratory research, although clinical and epidemiological research is also growing. Time spent in research should result in acquisition of an MD, PhD or equivalent, and publication of papers. The chances of achieving this depend on where and with whom the research is undertaken. Be sure that you are not being conned into being an extra pair of hands in clinic by a consultant who has no track record of supervising research! As it gets more difficult to get on to specialist registrar rotations, more intending nephrologists are going into research posts (not recognized for training) in the hope that this will help them to get on to the ladder later. An alternative is to obtain a LAT post, replacing someone who has taken time out of the rotation to do research. Both options carry a risk of never getting on to an specialist registrar rotation. There is currently a real danger that many specialist registrars will fail to find a consultant post. Such an expansion is needed but depends on individual trusts and health authorities recognizing the need for expansion.

Myth	Boffins, only interested in dialysis machines and renal tubular acidosis.
Reality	Old-fashioned clinical care is the most important aspect of the specialty: understanding glomerulonephritis, transplantation immunology, secondary hypertension and dialysis is taken as read.
Personality	More 'aggressive' than most physicians, but there's little room for those who can't talk to patients.
Best aspects	Wide range of disciplines involved; every patient is different.
Worst aspects	Hard work, demanding and complicated patients, frequent night calls. Dialysis and transplantation are expensive and the numbers of patients are growing, leading to constant conflict between maintaining standards and keeping within the budget.
Requirements	MRCP (PhD or MD often gained in the hope of improving job prospects)

Hours

Junior   Consultant

Numbers   230 posts (10–15 jobs per year)

Competitiveness

Stress

On-calls

Junior   Consultant

Salary   £50 000   £70 000   £100 000

For further information
Royal College of Physicians
11 St Andrew's Place
Regent's Park
London NW1 4LE
Tel: 020 7935 1174
Fax: 020 7487 5218
Website: www.rcplondon.ac.uk

119

Respiratory medicine

Specialists in respiratory (chest) medicine, like those in several other specialties, actually train in two specialties: their own and the much broader specialty, general internal medicine. This trains them to deal with a wide range of emergency medical conditions (heart attacks, strokes, severe infections, etc.) and equips them to take part in the 'on-take' rota which provides 24 hour-a-day cover for patients arriving at the hospital in emergencies. Almost all chest physicians in Britain practise in this way and most major hospitals have a chest physician on the staff who takes part in this general medical emergency rota. This makes the specialty attractive to young doctors. The jobs are interesting and there are plenty of them.

Respiratory medicine also has a strong academic tradition. Many of the tests and measurements which are used on patients are essentially physiological and there are a sizeable number of academic career opportunities.

Respiratory medicine has changed enormously in recent years. Technical advances include major improvements in our ability to look at the lung (e.g. by special X-ray and other methods), to look inside and take samples from the lung (by fibre-optic bronchoscopy and thoracoscopy) and to measure the function of the lung. At the same time, treatment for many lung diseases (such as asthma, pneumonia and tuberculosis) has improved immensely and the spectrum of lung diseases has expanded. All this makes respiratory medicine a growing, interesting and rapidly evolving specialty.

The training programme is similar to that in several other medical specialties. The SHO will be working in the wards and clinics, and studying (during study leave and spare time) for the MRCP. Specialist training has been amalgamated into the new specialist registrar grade which lasts five years and, if it progresses satisfactorily, ends with the award of a CCST in general internal medicine and respiratory medicine. This allows the specialist registrar to apply for consultant posts which will usually be held until retirement.

Once in a consultant post he or she will look after general medical and respiratory patients in the wards and clinics, take part in and supervise the training of junior staff and take responsibility for running the specialist respiratory service, including its patient testing facilities and laboratories. The work will involve collaborating with many other specialists, for example, radiologists, pathologists and surgeons, and with GPs, nursing and laboratory staff, physiotherapists, social workers and secretarial and clerical staff. The consultant will have to be available out-of-hours as well as during the day to advise on or see very ill or complicated patients, particularly on the on-take days. In consultant posts at teaching hospitals there will be student teaching and research to add to this list. And, of course, there are opportunities to get involved in the running of the hospital service. Some people like this and others hate it, but it is difficult to avoid.

Chest physicians are busy doctors with interests that range widely throughout medicine and make them central to the hospital service. Their specialty is growing, technical and science-based. In addition, it involves the ability to counsel and care for patients with chronic and fatal illness and a willingness to keep up in a changing specialty.

Myth	Old-fashioned group of wrinklies who shuffle round TB sanatoriums waving their stethoscopes impressively.
Reality	A hard working and rewarding hospital specialty which calls for technical skills, humanity and a wide range of medical knowledge.
Personality	Practical; interested in people; good communicators; not afraid of hard work and manual skills; technically literate.
Best aspects	Being at the centre of things; interesting and developing specialty; much human contact and hands-on work.
Worst aspects	Demanding training; dealing with lung cancer and bronchitis patients who won't stop smoking.
Requirements	MRCP (and MD/PhD for academic centres)

Hours

Junior   Consultant

Numbers 395 posts (9% are women)

Competitiveness

Stress

On-calls

Junior   Consultant

Salary £50 000   £70 000   £90000

For further information	**British Thoracic Society** 1 St Andrew's Place London NW1 4LB Tel: 020 7486 7766

Public health medicine

On taking up public health medicine you are concerned with the health of groups of people. What this means in practice is that you gather information about populations and set about devising policies for dealing with their health problems in the best way possible, combining prevention, treatment and care, and get them accepted and implemented. However, you do give up direct patient contact and involvement with individual cases. You do not wear a white coat, and only part of your time is spent with other health professionals; you may spend a lot of time with health service managers.

This is not, therefore, a job for those who need the satisfaction of patient contact. However, for those who want to control events rather than being at their mercy, and who want to shape the future, this is the place to be.

Once in the specialty, there are a lot of different areas to work in. Most of those in this specialty work with health authorities and currently their role is to assess the needs of the population and to develop effective strategies for the provision of services in conjunction with hospitals, general practice and community services. Some work only in the field of communicable disease control. However, many work outside this environment in regional offices, government departments and academic departments on a range of issues such as screening policies, cancer registration, manpower planning and epidemiological and health services research.

Pay is the same as in the NHS, the Civil Service or universities but in general the job is not as secure as in clinical medicine. This is mainly because of administrative change, but it is not unknown for those not considered to be pulling their weight by management to be eased out. Apart from those involved with communicable disease control, there is little on-call but the hours are still fairly long with evening and weekend work quite usual. It is not a job for the morbidly sensitive, since one of the functions of the jobs is the resolution of conflict with workable solutions, and it is difficult to do this and be loved by all.

The quality of those entering the specialty is high. You must have at least three years of good quality training after qualification, and a postgraduate diploma such as MRCGP or MRCP would improve your chances of selection. There has always been a unified training grade, and assuming that you obtain the public health medicine diploma, MFPHM, you are fairly sure of a stimulating job that will change throughout your career in the light of new challenges.

Myth	Related more to the Pay Corps than to the SAS.
Reality	More like Intelligence, with opportunities to shape the future of medicine.
Personality	Thick-skinned (this comes with practice). Able to cope with uncertainty.
Best aspects	Constant variety and challenge.
Worst aspects	Being affected by political whim.
Requirements	MFPHM, although other postgraduate qualifications an advantage.

Hours

Junior   Consultant

Numbers   871 posts   38% are women (602 NHS only)

Competitiveness

Stress

On-calls

Junior   Consultant

Salary

£min   £av   £max

£50000   £60 000   £70 000

For further information	**Faculty of Public Health Medicine** Royal College of Physicians 4 St Andrew's Place London NW1 4LB Tel: 020 7935 0243 Fax: 020 7224 6973

Musculoskeletal medicine

Undergraduate and postgraduate teaching of the treatment and rehabilitation of soft tissue injuries is growing in popularity rapidly, but is still extremely limited. This field of interest traditionally falls between the realms of orthopaedic surgery and rheumatology. However, there are those in the medical profession who are interested in the medical side of orthopaedics and the management of those injuries/conditions not requiring surgery or demonstrating any rheumatological disorder. Previously known as physical medicine and rehabilitation and occasionally referred to as orthopaedic medicine, this area is now called musculoskeletal medicine.

The British Institute of Musculoskeletal medicine (BIMM) was established in 1992 and runs a diploma course that was set up by the Society of Apothecaries in London. The BIMM is interested in sports medicine, osteopathic treatment, injection techniques, physiotherapy modalities and the many types of manipulation.

The requirements to become specialized in this subject may appear vague. The individual requires precise skills in diagnosis of soft tissue lesions. Palpation and further examination skills are far superior to those obtained at medical school (how many of us as an undergraduate were taught how to palpate for areas of hypertonia or scar tissue in a hamstring injury, or the degree of passive movement of L4 on L5 compared with that of L5 on S1?). The skill of injection techniques may then be learned as precise palpation/knowledge of surface anatomy is needed to locate 'the spot'. Cortisone, for example, is only effective if put into the inflamed tissue. The above diploma course will confirm specialist training, and this will be further established once the Royal Colleges have created a separate faculty and examination structure. The present Royal College qualification is useful to avoid red tape, but will provide few of the skills required for this specialty.

Relevant junior doctor experience should be in orthopaedics, rheumatology, casualty, general medicine and a taste of general practice (where over 30% of patients are presenting with musculoskeletal complaints that may not lead to mortality but represent the largest portion of morbidity). As more posts in musculoskeletal medicine crop up around the country, exposure to their teaching expertise will become more available on hospital rotations.

Rehabilitation after a soft tissue injury is most prevalent in the exercising population and therefore the timing of modalities of treatment is important (this will differ depending on patients, their chosen sports and their degree of motivation). The specialist will treat the acute injury, assist restoration of function as soon as possible, prevent re-injury, provide an exercise prescription to maintain fitness during recovery (e.g. swimming with a pool buoy or cycling with one leg) and have the ability to assess the success of the treatment (i.e. laboratory work with muscle, serological and physiological tests).

The doctor therefore works in a multidisciplinary environment with a wide range of patients from the international athlete to the chronic low-back pain sufferer. The work is rewarding as the service is supplying a demand that has been present for some time.

Our colleagues around the world are at various stages of creating and progressing this specialty. FIMM is the global organization that sets standards. The European Association of Musculoskeletal Medicine has established the specialty on a formal basis in four countries and is expanding. So the specialisms of orthopaedics and rheumatology will no longer be able to prevent the growth of this field of medicine which addresses non-surgical and non-inflammatory orthopaedic problems.

Myth	Buttock massagers who inject anything that moves.
Reality	Pioneers because of their attempts to re-establish a specialty that disappeared in the 1950s. Growing interest in this field which has close links with sports medicine.
Personality	Varied, from the sports enthusiast who wants to get out there on to the pitch, to the serious medical manipulator who looks beyond the realms of traditional (?dated) medical science
Best aspects	Patient contact is second to none. Learn new and varied skills where your advice, help and assistance will be required by friends and colleagues at most social functions ('I've had this pain just over my right shoulder for 6 months and all the doctor gives me is tablets. What do you think?')
Worst aspects	Royal Colleges are being slow to create separate specialties in both this and sports medicine. Training at most levels is difficult to find. Some not-so-nice buttocks to massage.
Requirements	Diploma of musculoskeletal medicine (or an equivalent), plus relevant experience (details of which are available from the address below).

Hours

Junior   Consultant

Numbers	Seven specialist NHS posts at present with many more in the pipeline. Most practitioners are therefore in private practice.
Competitiveness	None (there are not enough to go round)

Stress

On-calls

Junior   Consultant

Salary

£50 000   £60 000   £90 000

For further information	**British Institute of Musculoskeletal Medicine** 34 The Avenue Watford Herts WD1 3NS Tel/Fax: 01923 220999 Website: www.bimm.org.uk

125

Rheumatology

The specialty of rheumatology is concerned with the management and treatment of disorders of the musculoskeletal system. The specialty has changed dramatically over the last 30 years from a fringe specialty linked to the department of physiotherapy (often called the department of physical medicine) to a mainstream subspecialty within general medicine. This metamorphosis is due largely to the recognition that many of the disorders affecting the musculoskeletal system are in fact conditions that also affect many other organ systems. Research into many of these autoimmune disorders has at times led the way within the clinical specialties in helping to understand the basic mechanisms of our immune system.

Rheumatology rarely has a major place in the undergraduate curriculum, with priority of teaching often placed on more acute specialties such as cardiology. Many rheumatologists only had sufficient exposure to spark of their interest in the specialty at a postgraduate level, often as an SHO. This situation has improved in recent years with rheumatology being taught in the context of 'musculoskeletal disorders' along with orthopaedics.

A sound background in general (internal) medicine is always needed for general professional training prior to subspecialization in rheumatology. During these two years it is vitally important to take and succeed in passing Parts I and II of the MRCP examination, in order to proceed to a registrar post.

Higher training in rheumatology can be divided into four main career paths: (i) clinical rheumatology alone; (ii) dual specialization with general medicine; (iii) academic rheumatology; and (iv) dual specialization with rehabilitation. The majority of consultant posts are in clinical rheumatology alone. Within the new specialist registrar grade, rotations last either four (single specialization) or five (dual specialization) years, reflecting these different career endpoints. Training in rehabilitation now has a separate career path and these days posts are rarely combined with rheumatology.

A period of time in research is generally expected, although trainees can obtain consultant posts, particularly in district general hospitals without obtaining a higher degree (MD/PhD).

Rheumatologists work closely with other disciplines including orthopaedic surgeons, occupational therapists, physiotherapists and podiatrists. It is a common misconception, amongst both the general public and the medical profession itself, that arthritis is a condition that only affects old people. Many types of arthritis, for which we have treatment, affect young adults and children. However, someone wishing to specialize in rheumatology has to be prepared to see both the interesting disorders, such as the inflammatory connective tissue disorders, and the far more common complaints, such as back pain, for which we have little scientific understanding and poorly effective treatments.

New treatments, particularly monoclonal antibodies produced by bioengineering techniques, offer exciting times ahead for both rheumatologists and their patients.

Myth	Doctors looking after patients with chronic incurable disorders, seeing no-one but old people and moaning minnies.
Reality	A mixture of opportunities from highbrow complex immunologically orientated posts to those interested in the workings and frailties of the human skeleton. Exciting future treatment possibilities derived from basic research for patients with arthritis.
Personality	Extremely varied, from patient-phobic lymphocyte-loving scientist to patient, caring, good listeners.
Best aspects	Varied conditions to treat, from potentially fatal multisystem connective tissue disorders to regional musculoskeletal complaints including sports injuries. Long-term contact with many patients often very rewarding.
Worst aspects	Lack of effective treatments to offer for certain conditions—and the same patients keep coming back!
Requirements	MRCP (MD/PhD for jobs in major centres)

Hours

Junior   Consultant

Numbers 370 posts (10–20 per year) 20% are women

Competitiveness

Stress

On-calls

Junior   Consultant

Salary

£50 000   £65 000   £150000

For further information	**The British Society for Rheumatology** 41 Eagle Street London WC1R 4AR Tel: 020 7242 3313 Fax: 020 7242 3277 Website: www.rheumatology.org.uk	**Royal College of Physicians** 11 St Andrew's Place Regent's Park London NW1 4LE Tel: 020 7935 1174 Fax 020 7487 5218

Sports medicine

This specialty sounds sexy but it isn't. For a start, there is no career structure. Secondly, if you do it you are likely to lose your family because you are spending all the normal social hours looking after teams and athletes, and the excitement of a seat on the bench can very rapidly diminish on a freezing cold, wet day, when there is no cover and you have got to sew up the heads of opposing rugby front rows.

Despite that, there is a group of doctors in this country determined to do sports medicine, either on its own or as part of another job. For the main part, that other job is in general practice although one or two other specialities are involved.

The types of sports medicine doctors are going to reflect the types of athletes. There are a very large number of people with an interest in sports medicine who usually do one session a week in their general practice surgery who look after 'recreational' athletes, possibly including local meetings. He or she should have a diploma in sports medicine. That diploma can be achieved full time at the course at the London Hospital Medical College (a University of London award) or part-time through the Bath distance-learning course, leading to an examination by the Royal Colleges of Surgeons in Scotland or the Worshipful Society of Apothecaries in London.

For the next level of sport (e.g. a professional soccer club), there should be the next level of expertise. Again, the doctor will be a primary care physician but with a much greater commitment to sports medicine represented by an MSc now available at Nottingham or the London Hospital Medical College. Clearly, far more time has to be committed and a significant component of continuing medical education is important.

At the highest level, for the top class athlete, there should be top class sports physicians. There is a group of doctors already in this country who do nothing else and they provide a very good service. It is hoped that the structure in sports medicine will evolve, so that some sort of collegiate function will exist to offer these doctors at the pinnacle of the profession a fellowship reflecting their commitment to the athlete at the highest level.

Remuneration is very much at the rates of a principal in general practice. However, for those who wish to do this job exclusively, it is a hand-to-mouth existence, involving a number of contracts with clubs, possibly national squads or associations, and a private practice. In the longer term I hope to see the title changed to 'exercise and sports injury medicine', reflecting the preventive medicine role, but I still feel, for the foreseeable future, it will be a special interest within general practice for the majority and a fraught lifestyle for the minority who choose to do this work full-time.

The essential skills are obviously enhanced knowledge of exercise physiology, testing, etc.; slightly less obvious requirements are an ability to get on with and talk the same language as the athletes you are treating and an exceedingly understanding family.

Myth	Get to see all the big games, treat high-profile players and get appropriate recognition.
Reality	You are always underground in a smelly room. You miss the games. No-one has heard of 98% of the people you treat.
Personality	You must be a communicator and motivator. You have to build trust with an athlete like no other branch of medicine (they are not actually ill).
Best aspects	Get to the top and you'll have a seat in the director's box, go to the Olympics, and treat highly motivated, fit people with good back-up resources.
Worst aspects	Sports medicine politics are terrible and no-one agrees about anything. You work long hours in muddy corners. There is no career structure.
Requirements	Diploma not yet validated. One year postgraduate MSc is best, but there is no European agreement.
Hours	your athlete will find you, day or night, where ever you are
Numbers	Five full-time NHS posts; most are part-time **30%** are women
Competitiveness	
Stress	
On-calls	(see note under 'hours')
Salary	£35 000 £60 000 £100 000
For further information	There is no recognized 'body' For advice you can try: **The Academic Department of Sports Medicine,** St Bart's and the Royal London Hospital School of Medicine and Dentistry Queen Mary and Westfield College London E1 4DG

Spinal cord injury

As a recently qualified doctor, a career in 'spinal injuries' is not one that readily springs to mind, possibly because it is one of the smaller specialties, but also because there is often no formal teaching at undergraduate level. It is probably assumed that it is a branch of neurosurgery or orthopaedics, but accreditation is actually under 'rehabilitation medicine'.

The speciality is correctly called 'spinal cord injury' (SCI), a term now recognized by the Specialist Advisory Committee in Rehabilitation Medicine. The 11 spinal injuries units in Britain provide a comprehensive regional or supraregional service (acute and follow-up), primarily for people with spinal injuries and cord damage—paraplegia and tetraplegia. Ten to fifteen per cent of patients are paralysed as a result of medical conditions (e.g. spinal artery thrombosis, tumours or infection).

This is much more of a consultant-led service than most specialities and the management of SCI requires a multidisciplinary team approach. This is led by consultants in spinal injuries and involves doctors, nurses, therapists, social workers and clinical psychologists, and often specialists from other fields such as urology, orthopaedics, general medicine, general surgery, plastic surgery, neurology, neurosurgery and psychiatry. The doctor specializing in spinal injuries therefore needs to have a broad general knowledge, and someone coming from almost any medical or surgical background will almost certainly have something to offer even when new to the subject. There are opportunities to develop special interests (e.g. the management of the neuropathic bladder or assisted fertility), depending on the person's previous experience. Although surgeons are at present in the majority, about a third of consultants are physicians, reflecting the wide nature of the specialty.

It is advisable to have good grounding at SHO level in general medicine, general surgery, accident and emergency medicine, and orthopaedics, before embarking on a career in spinal injuries. Specialist registrar training is four years with at least two years spent in a spinal injuries unit. It must be emphasized that someone accredited in rehabilitation who has only spent three months in a spinal injuries unit will not have the necessary expertise to deal with the unique mixture of acute and chronic multisystem pathology seen in SCI patients. A specialist registrar will need to gain experience in intensive care because, as resuscitation techniques at the scene of accidents have improved, more patients are surviving with complex problems and/or high tetraplegia, and an increasing number of these are requiring short- or long-term ventilation.

Apart from the minority of SCI patients who make a complete recovery, most other patients are followed up for life. It is therefore vital in this speciality that doctors must be able to relate well to people: patients, families and carers, as well as health workers in the community. A holistic approach is certainly necessary. Although the 'cure rate' may be low, it is easy to underestimate the inner strengths of people with SCI. To be able to play a central role in their rehabilitation following such a devastating injury and to see them achieving a surprisingly high quality of life and often a remarkable degree of independence can be uniquely satisfying.

Myth	Making the paralysed walk.
Reality	Only a minority of patients recover sufficiently to walk. The consultant is head of a multidisciplinary team involved in the emergency, acute and more long-term aspect of paraplegia and tetraplegia.
Personality	Must be able to work in a team and relate well to relatives, patients and staff.
Best aspects	A diversifying field with considerable opportunities for research. Surprisingly wide variety of medicine. Spinal injuries units tend to have a very supportive, relaxed and friendly atmosphere.
Worst aspects	Frustrations of having a patient well rehabilitated, but whose discharge home is delayed by a lack of community care and suitable accommodation.
Requirements	MRCS or MRCP

Hours

Junior   Consultant

Numbers   21 posts   10% are women

Competitiveness

Stress

On-calls

Junior   Consultant

Salary

£50 000   £70 000   £120 000

For further information	**Specialist Advisory Committee in Rehabilitation Medicine** Royal College of Physicians 11 St Andrew's Place Regents Park London NW1 4LE Tel: 020 7935 1174 Fax: 020 7487 5218

Accident and emergency: career pathway

Duration

1 year

3–5 years

4–5 years

~30 years

EXAM OR COURSE
Medical college Finals

Provisionally registered House Officer

Senior House Officer in a variety of fields

EXAM OR COURSE
MRCS(A&E)Ed / MRCS / MRCP / Primary FRCA

Post membership Senior House Officer

Non-career grades
(Posts outside the training hierachy)

Specialist Registrar

EXAM OR COURSE
MSc/Research

EXAM OR COURSE
FFAEM

Award of CCST

Time abroad

Consultant

Key:

Compulsory route

Optional route

Whilst theoretically possible to apply for an A&E SpR post with 2 years experience in Medicine, Surgery or Anaesthetics and that Colleges exam, given that A&E is getting increasingly competetive, candidates are expected to show a breadth of SHO training suitable for the inevitable variety of A&E.

The requirements for the MRCS(A&E)Ed exam are 1 years experience in each of medicine, surgery and A&E. This can include housejobs. There is no specific part 1 for this exam – one can take the MRCP, MRCS OR FRCA first part and then the A&E part 2. Many A&E SpRs (and consultants) have more than one exam.

Accident and emergency medicine

Accident and emergency medicine

Accident and Emergency (A&E) is a young, rapidly expanding hospital specialty. It has shrugged off its (slightly unfair) historical label of being staffed by failed or uninterested surgeons and is now an attractive option for dynamic medical graduates.

A&E departments receive patients with an almost limitless range of emergency problems. The A&E doctor therefore requires a good and broad-based medical knowledge. Perhaps more important, however, is the possession of common sense, combined with considerable tact and patience. The work is constantly challenging and interesting. Having to respond quickly to difficult situations and make critical decisions under pressure is inevitably stressful, but is also hugely rewarding.

The specialty is rapidly becoming more competitive. The critical step in pursuing a career in A&E is to obtain a five-year specialist registrar post. The minimum requirement is to gain some experience in A&E and one or more other hospital specialties and to acquire a postgraduate qualification. A&E is unusual in that it can be entered from a variety of different backgrounds: medicine, surgery or anaesthetics. It is also possible to train specifically for A&E at SHO level. It is now hard to get a specialist registrar post without breadth of posts on the CV and there are now SHO rotations aimed at meeting the requirements of the MRCS(A&E) exam run by the Royal College of Surgeons of Edinburgh.

The emphasis of specialist registrar training in A&E is directed towards practical issues. The newly established Faculty of A&E Medicine (FAEM) is responsible for coordinating training and research within the specialty. Trainees are helped to acquire the skills needed to become competent in managing the wide range of emergency conditions commonly seen, especially those that are life-threatening. In addition, management training and secondments to an exciting and unusually wide variety of other specialties are arranged and tailored according to individual needs. Although an MD or other higher research degree is not required, research is strongly encouraged and can count towards accreditation. Towards the end of the training period there is an 'exit' examination organized by the Faculty. Successful negotiation of this results in acquisition of Fellowship of the Faculty of Accident and Emergency Medicine (FFAEM). There then follows the difficult, but exciting, task of choosing and applying for a consultant post.

Work as a consultant in A&E is centred around providing the best possible service for patients. Considering the heavy demand on A&E services and the current staffing structure, it is inevitable that the majority of patients will continue to be seen by non-consultant-grade staff. A critical part of the A&E consultant's role is therefore to establish a safe and efficient system for patient care; this results in a significant proportion of time spent teaching. It is also important to coordinate a highly motivated multidisciplinary team. Nurses are taking on an increasing diversity of roles in A&E; emergency nurse practitioners (ENPs) are well established in many sites. It is an exciting time to be in such a revitalized and evolving specialty.

As a consultant there is potential to subspecialize. Established fields include areas as diverse as paediatric A&E, sports medicine, hand injuries, expedition medicine, prehospital care and tele-medicine.

Myth	Just watch *ER*—a glamorous job which involves saving a life every five minutes.
Reality	Hard work, unpredictable in nature, but constantly interesting and frequently rewarding.
Personality	Leadership skills are helpful, common sense essential
Best aspects	Arguably the most varied hospital job—you do occasionally 'save a life'.
Worst aspects	The hours are inherently antisocial. A significant proportion of patients are aggressive and/or heavily under the influence of alcohol/drugs. Opportunities to follow up patients long-term are limited.
Requirements	Entry via MRCS, MRCS(A&E), MRCP or FRCA. Exit via FFAEM

Hours

Junior   to   depending on set-up
           Consultant

Numbers   450 posts rising at 25 per year   16% are women

Competitiveness

but getting more competitive

Stress

On-calls   fixed shifts

Junior   Consultant

Salary

£50 000   £75 000   £120 000

For further information

Faculty of Accident and Emergency Medicine
Royal College of Surgeons of England
35–43 Lincoln's Inn Fields
London WC2A 3PN
Tel: 020 7405 7071
Fax: 020 7405 0318

Paediatrics: career pathway

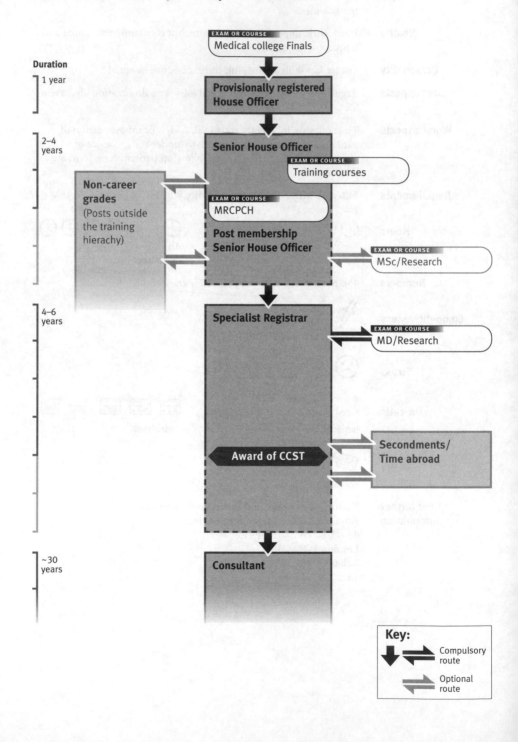

Duration

1 year

2–4 years

4–6 years

~30 years

EXAM OR COURSE
Medical college Finals

Provisionally registered House Officer

Senior House Officer

EXAM OR COURSE
Training courses

Non-career grades
(Posts outside the training hierachy)

EXAM OR COURSE
MRCPCH

Post membership Senior House Officer

EXAM OR COURSE
MSc/Research

Specialist Registrar

EXAM OR COURSE
MD/Research

Award of CCST

Secondments/ Time abroad

Consultant

Key:

Compulsory route

Optional route

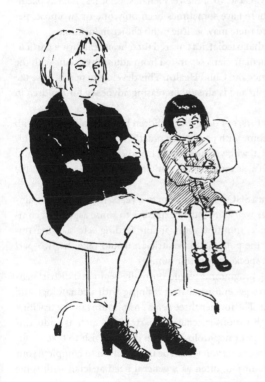
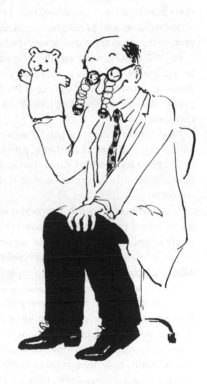

CHAPTER 8
Paediatrics

Most paediatricians are general physicians to infants, children and adolescents or are working as community paediatricians for the same age range. A smaller number of paediatricians become very specialized both in hospital or in a community setting and may, for example, concentrate entirely on cardiology, neurology, nephrology, or physical and mental disability.

Hospital-based paediatrics can vary enormously depending, for example, on whether the post is in a small district general hospital or in a large teaching hospital. In the district general hospital the paediatrician will require skills and expertise in the whole range of subspecialties. However, in a large teaching hospital, there will often be colleagues in subspecialties and even the general paediatrician may be expected to develop subspecialty interests as well.

Paediatrics has become increasingly 'user friendly' for women graduates and those who may wish to train part-time. Competition for paediatric consultant posts in the future is difficult to predict. With the rapid expansion of community paediatrics over the ten years between 1985 and 1995, there have been fewer candidates than jobs available. In some very small specialties, such as paediatric cardiology and paediatric neurology, there have sometimes been only one or two posts per year, so the competition can be very severe and there may be little or no choice in location.

In 1997, it was finally formally recognized that paediatrics covered total healthcare for a particular age group (25% of the population) and paediatricians separated from adult physicians with the development of the Royal College of Paediatrics and Child Health. This development will raise the profile of paediatricians as a professional group and is already increasing advocacy for children in their own right.

Paediatricians have to be good communicators, not only with children but (less obviously) with young adults. Almost all paediatric patients come with parents. In practice, most of the communication that a paediatrician carries out is, in fact, with young women (mothers). Paediatricians also have a major role in communicating with GPs, schools, social workers and other agencies in the community.

The training of a paediatrician begins with an SHO programme of two years, to get a broad training in general paediatrics with neonatology as well as adequate exposure to some aspects of community paediatrics, such as child surveillance, immunization, infant feeding, etc. During this two-year rotation it would be expected that the potential paediatrician would take the two-part MRCPCH exam, allowing them to apply for a specialist registrar number.

At this stage, the specialist registrar training programme would normally begin in a district general hospital with two years of comprehensive general paediatric training with neonatology and then a rotation into a larger teaching hospital. The further three years (minimum) in the teaching hospital would also include rotations through various specialist departments, such as endocrinology, diabetes, respiratory medicine, neurology or nephrology. If you did not wish to take a subspecialization any further, at the end of the three years you would be in a position to complete your training programme and apply for a consultant job, often as a general paediatrician with some specialty interest that has been reflected in your earlier training.

For specialty training at a tertiary level you could put your training programme 'on hold' while you did a year or two of research or specialist training experience, for example in another country. You might also choose at this point to go into one of the very specialist subspecialties such as neurology or cardiology which would add one to three years more to the specialist registrar training for CCST recognition in addition to the CCST for general paediatrics.

Myth	Big kids swinging tiny stethoscopes and wearing Disney ties.
Reality	All specialties relating to growth and development. Patients from 24 weeks' gestation to over 24 years. Most paediatricians are general physicians to children and often have a subspecialty interest.
Personality	Sense of humour mandatory. Calm and approachable.
Best aspects	Great variety; high cure rate in most areas. Flexible training options are well established.
Worst aspects	Can have high emotional content—failure can be catastrophic. Limited scope for private practice. Babies don't know the difference between night and day!
Requirements	MRCPCH

Hours

Junior 🕐🕐🕐🕐🕐   Consultant 🕐🕐🕐🕐🕐

Numbers 1200 posts   35% are women

Competitiveness 🗡🗡🗡🗡🗡

Stress ☹☹☹☹☹

On-calls

Junior 📟📟📟📟📟   Consultant 📟📟📟📟📟

Salary

£min £50 000   £av £68 000   £max £110 000

For further information	**Royal College of Paediatrics and Child Health** 50 Hallum Street London W1N 6DE Tel: 020 7307 5600 Fax: 020 7307 5601 Website: www.rcph.ac.uk

CHAPTER 9

Diagnostic and interventional radiology

Diagnostic and interventional radiology

Clinical radiology and imaging are concerned with finding out what is wrong with patients and requires interaction with other clinicians in their management. Increasingly, with interventional procedures, radiologists are more directly involved in treatment. Doctors in radiology now divide their time between performing diagnostic and therapeutic procedures on patients (e.g. barium studies, ultrasound, arteriography or guided biopsy) and interpreting X-ray films or other images obtained by radiographers or technicians working under their guidance. The reports issued and the subsequent discussions increasingly form an important interaction with colleagues in the bed-holding specialties and with GPs to work out how to solve clinical problems. Radiologists need to advise on the choice of imaging methods and do their best to produce effective diagnostic results whilst minimizing the exposure of patients to ionizing radiation.

Over the last 25 years the role of the radiologist has expanded in parallel with major developments in imaging technology, with the introduction of ultrasound, computed tomography (CT) and magnetic resonance imaging (MRI). Although the newer approaches are now widely used, plain radiography and contrast examinations such as barium studies and intravenous urograms still play an important role. The traditional methods have not been entirely superseded by the new technologies; rather, their use has become increasingly specific for the investigation of particular clinical problems. The increasing range and complexity of imaging techniques means that few physicians and surgeons manage to maintain a breadth of knowledge about the available methods, so they have become more and more dependent on the focused expertise of the radiologist.

Radiologists investigate everybody else's patients. Interaction with doctors in other specialties is an important part of everyday life and it helps for the radiologist to have an encyclopaedic knowledge of clinical medicine, pathology and medical and surgical therapy, which is why most appointment committees for radiology training schemes are looking for doctors who have had broad experience before entering radiology. A firm grasp of imaging technology is essential, but anyone who thinks machines are more fun than people should seek an alternative line of work.

The other major development in the last 25 years is the increasing number of therapeutic procedures performed by radiologists as an alternative to surgery, often when surgery cannot be successfully or safely used. There is a broad spectrum of interventional procedures, but increasingly the interventional radiologist is becoming more specialized, tending to work within one body system, e.g. vascular or urological. This allows a close working relationship with colleagues in the bed-holding specialties and the radiologist can become integrated within the clinical team. This certainly occurs in many teaching hospitals where each of several radiologists may practise interventional procedures within their own clinical subspecialty. In district general hospitals, interventional radiologists are likely to perform a wider range of procedures. Thus, as for interpretive or diagnostic radiologists, the pattern of work for interventionalists varies considerably from place to place allowing choice to suit the individual. For many individuals interventional radiology is more appealing, and may be more rewarding, than reporting piles of routine films, but most of these procedures are alternatives to surgery and carry with them significant risks and the possibility of unpleasant complications. The intervention radiologist needs not only to be good with his/her hands, but also to have the mental stamina to cope with the tensions of surgical-type procedures and the physical stamina to work standing in a lead coat for hours on end. Interventional radiology also requires a continuing commitment, with an increasing proportion of out-of-hours working.

Training and accreditation in the UK are controlled by the Royal College of Radiologists.

Radiology: career pathway

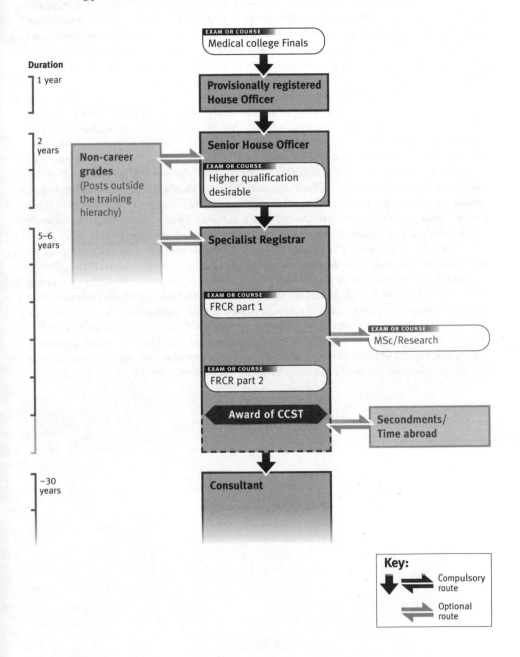

Duration

EXAM OR COURSE
Medical college Finals

1 year

Provisionally registered House Officer

2 years

Non-career grades
(Posts outside the training hierachy)

Senior House Officer

EXAM OR COURSE
Higher qualification desirable

5–6 years

Specialist Registrar

EXAM OR COURSE
FRCR part 1

EXAM OR COURSE
MSc/Research

EXAM OR COURSE
FRCR part 2

Award of CCST

Secondments/ Time abroad

~30 years

Consultant

Key:

Compulsory route

Optional route

Accreditation follows five years of fairly well defined full-time training in an approved department which may include a short period spent on research. After achieving success at the FRCR examination, a CCST is granted. The period of training may be extended by a further year for subspecialty training in some areas such as neuroradiology or interventional radiology. Overseas experience can only be obtained during this period if it is obtained in recognized departments and in countries with reciprocal recognition of training. Some radiologists choose to do overseas Fellowships following completion of UK training to improve their experience—and their CV!

Most of the training programmes (which exist in all the UK cities with medical schools) start with an annual intake of trainees in September or October, with interviews in the preceding January or February, with a view to trainees undertaking Part I of the FRCR examination in the following May. The Part I examination covers radiographic and radiological techniques, anatomy and physics relevant to radiology. There is a substantial taught element in the first year but most of the remainder of the training is an apprenticeship in the various subspecialties within radiology. The Part II of the FRCR is now split into two parts, the first being an MCQ paper and the second a film-reading examination and orals. A good candidate should expect to complete this around the end of their third year or beginning of their fourth year. On-call work is an essential part of the training, trainees work under consultant supervision with increasing independence as their seniority and experience grow.

Radiology is still a shortage specialty and one that continues to expand. Consultant posts can be very different from each other depending upon the location, type of hospital, and type of work involved. To some degree, the range of activity can be tailored to the personality of the incumbent so there is room for the thoughtful and intense (reading mammography films), the practical extrovert (intervention procedures) and the technical whizzkid (MRI). Most consultants will be able to find a rewarding balance between cognitive and manipulative activity depending upon their preference. Contact with patients is frequent but usually brief and episodic. Nonetheless, the specialty is called clinical radiology for good reason: clinical radiologists are well trained doctors first of all, who subsequently become specialists in imaging, diagnosis and interventional procedures.

Myth	Bad-tempered introverts who prefer to be left alone in dark rooms.
Reality	Clinical detectives finding out what's wrong with patients and occasionally fixing it themselves; more usually facilitating medical or surgical treatment.
Personality	Fluency in communication helps. The range of tasks accommodates most types from the obsessive (reading piles of film) to the manic (thrombolysis at midnight).
Best aspects	Contact with patients is mostly in acute episodes; there is lots of scope for technical innovation; collaboration with a wide range of clinical specialties.
Worst aspects	Getting barium—or worse—on your suede shoes. Dealing with colleagues in other specialties who know everything.
Requirements	FRCR or equivalent overseas qualification

Hours

Junior   Consultant

Numbers   1287 posts   24% are women

Competitiveness

Stress

On-calls

Junior   Consultant

Salary

£50 000   £72 000   £100 000

For further information

Royal College of Radiologists
38 Portland Place
London W1 N 4JQ
Tel: 020 7636 4432
Fax: 020 7323 3100
Website: www.rcr.ac.uk

CHAPTER 10

Psychiatry

Overview

Mental health problems are common and account for a significant proportion of health service spending. Psychiatrists are usually one of the largest consultant groups in most districts but, because they are often based away from the general hospital, may have a relatively low impact on students and on trainees outside their discipline. Because of this low profile and because undergraduate psychiatry teaching often focuses on adult psychiatry, misconceptions about psychiatry are rife. The popular image of the bearded man with a German accent listening to a patient lying prone on a couch is about as far from the truth as it is possible to get!

In fact, psychiatry can be one of the most stimulating, interesting and rewarding fields in medicine. Psychiatrists, like specialists in other medical disciplines, are doctors first and specialists second. Their training in medicine, the biological neurosciences, developmental psychology and sociology gives them a unique perspective on patients' problems. Psychiatric problems are complex and trying to make sense of the apparently incomprehensible (to the lay public) problems that may present is an intellectual challenge. Psychiatrists require good communication and listening skills, patience, a capacity to form close working relationships with their patients and an inquisitive, thoughtful and creative disposition.

Psychiatry is at least as clinically effective as other medical disciplines, and even with problems where complete resolution is not possible, significant improvements in quality of life can often be achieved. However, the work is demanding and can be emotionally stressful—psychiatrists need to strike a balance between maintaining the distance necessary to provide useful insights into difficult behaviour and the compassion and sensitivity needed to engage patients and their families in treatment.

Psychiatric training is well organized compared with many other specialities, with detailed learning objectives at each stage of training. Trainees are involved at local and national level in both setting standards and objectives and in inspecting training schemes to ensure that standards are achieved. The Royal College places a strong emphasis on individual supervision as part of the training process and all trainees at whatever stage of training will receive a minimum of one hour of individual face-to-face supervision from their consultant each week.

Basic specialist training at SHO level is organized into rotational schemes. Part I of the membership examination (an MCQ test of knowledge and an assessment of clinical skills) can be taken after one year in either adult or old-age psychiatry. Following this the SHO spends a further two to three years rotating through other subspecialties before sitting Part II of the examination (MCQ, short notes, essay, critical appraisal skills and a second, more detailed, clinical assessment). All trainees must complete at least six months in either child and adolescent psychiatry or learning disability psychiatry. Up to one year of other relevant SHO experience (general practice, general medicine, paediatrics, etc.) can be counted towards the time needed before membership can be taken. SHOs are expected to attend a formal academic programme as part of preparation for the membership examination. This usually involves day release to a regional programme that in many areas leads to a Masters degree as well as providing preparation for the exam. In addition, all training schemes will put on a variety of local journal clubs, case presentations, research meetings, etc.

After successfully passing the membership examination, trainees apply for a specialist registrar post in the subspeciality of their choosing. In psychiatry there are separate 'Calman' trainings, each of which lasts a minimum of three years, in:

Psychiatry: career pathway

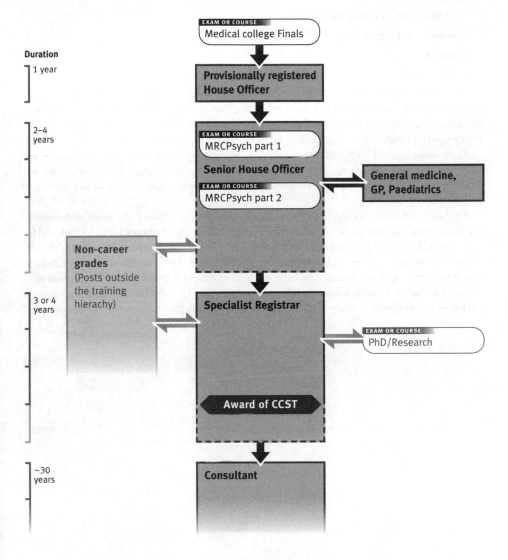

Duration

1 year

2–4 years

3 or 4 years

~30 years

EXAM OR COURSE
Medical college Finals

Provisionally registered House Officer

EXAM OR COURSE
MRCPsych part 1

Senior House Officer

EXAM OR COURSE
MRCPsych part 2

General medicine, GP, Paediatrics

Non-career grades
(Posts outside the training hierachy)

Specialist Registrar

EXAM OR COURSE
PhD/Research

Award of CCST

Consultant

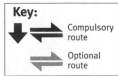

Key:

Compulsory route

Optional route

- adult psychiatry
- old-age psychiatry
- child and adolescent psychiatry
- learning disability psychiatry
- forensic psychiatry
- psychotherapy

In addition, within adult psychiatry it is possible to develop special interests in liaison psychiatry—the interface between physical disease and psychiatric problems and substance misuse psychiatry. Various combinations of the above trainings are also possible, for example forensic psychiatry and psychotherapy, although these take longer than the usual three years.

At specialist registrar level, some subspecialities continue the practice of expecting attendance at local academic programmes and all specialist registrars irrespective of specialism have one day per week of protected time for research—something not usually available in specialities outside of psychiatry.

Psychiatry remains a shortage specialty: there are more posts available at all levels than trainees to fill them. However, there are wide variations across the country and between subspecialties and for many posts there is still fierce competition. Trainees entering psychiatry should have little difficulty in finding jobs to suit them and in progressing to consultant level. Psychiatry attracts almost as many women as it does men, and women are well represented at the top of the profession at consultant and professorial levels. Psychiatry training is also very flexible and very supportive of part-time training, with as many as 20–30% of trainees working part-time in some subspecialties.

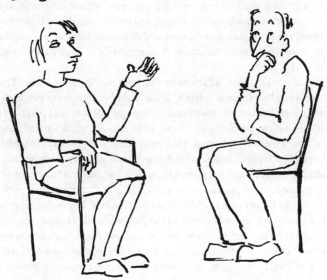

and can you remember when it was you FIRST thought of becoming a psychotherapist?

Adult psychiatry

Psychiatry is fascinating. There are no two ways about it. Of course, as a psychiatrist myself I may be a little biased—but an interest in the psyche is not confined to my psychiatric colleagues and me. Friends, family, plumbers, farmers, solicitors and many others, even including one's surgical colleagues, often harbour this fascination. It is difficult to comprehend why some doctors go off into less interesting areas of medicine!

As a psychiatrist you find yourself in a privileged position. Patients tell you their most personal and private concerns. They confide in you regarding what is troubling them. They may be hallucinating, suffering alarming delusions, unable to stop checking, uninhibited and grandiose or in the pit of depressive despair. They may be experiencing panic attacks or be referred to you because of chronic physical symptoms for which there is no apparent organic cause. The list of possibilities goes on and on. Access to the details of patients' psychological problems is not, however, a given right. It is achievable partly by virtue of the advanced training in communication and interviewing skills which you will have received and partly because, in psychiatry, we have more time (and the inclination) to ask and to listen.

Psychiatry is not an easy option. It can be emotionally draining and requires sustained concentration and thought regarding the problems you are presented with. Technological advances and increasingly effective treatments are actively sought and enthusiastically welcomed, but so far you can't send off a blood test or request a brain scan to differentiate between paranoid schizophrenia and a manic state or to diagnose somatization. You must rely in large part on your knowledge, experience and clinical acumen.

Not all psychiatrists working with 'adults of working age' are the same either. There are several well-established subspecialties to choose from. These include community psychiatry, addictions, forensic psychiatry, rehabilitation psychiatry and liaison (general hospital) psychiatry. Each has its own particular mix of patient problems and therapeutic approaches. An added area of interest in adult psychiatry is that of medicolegal issues. These may relate to the use of the Mental Health Act in clinical practice, specialist forensic issues or advising other healthcare professionals on aspects of common law and a patient's capacity to consent to, or to refuse, medical treatment.

The overriding theme in adult psychiatry is *variety*: variety of psychiatric conditions, investigations and treatments. The latter range from the biological (an ever-improving array of medications as well as modified electroconvulsive therapy) to the psychological (various approaches including cognitive behavioural therapy, interpersonal therapy and psychodynamic psychotherapy). Many psychiatrists also work in several different settings, from acute inpatient wards to day hospitals and community clinics. We work very closely with other members of a multidisciplinary team. Nurses, occupational therapists, social workers, psychologists and others combine to take an overall biopsychosocial (holistic) approach to dealing with the patient's problems. Psychiatry differs from many areas of medicine in that it has not become focused upon a single bodily system.

If you are interested in delving into what is troubling a person, and generating an effective way of helping them, psychiatry may be right up your street. The most important thing is to see its fascination. But then, how could you not?

Myth	An easy option. Only three or four conditions to deal with. Asylum doctors looking after only 'mad' people. Agents of social control, main purpose being to lock people up.
Reality	Very varied work. The challenge of generating a biopsychosocial understanding of the patient's problems and a multidisciplinary approach to management make this area interesting and enjoyable. Risk management and the nature of some patients' problems can be very demanding and emotionally draining.
Personality	A good communicator and team player. Enthusiastic and empathic.
Best aspects	Variety of psychiatric conditions, investigations, treatment options, research opportunities and possible subspecialization.
Worst aspects	A heavy workload with the possibility of burn-out (more so due to the increasing emphasis on risk management, especially of patients in the community).
Requirements	MRCPsych

Hours

Junior   Consultant

Numbers   1370 posts   23% are women

Competitiveness

Stress

On-calls

Junior   Consultant

Salary

£min   £av   £max

£55 000   £70 000   £100 000

For further information	**Royal College of Psychiatrists** 17 Belgrave Square London SW1X 8PG Tel: 020 7235 2351 Fax: 020 7245 1231 Website: www.rcpsych.ac.uk

Child and adolescent psychiatry

This is a growing subspecialty. Child mental health is a priority area for Government and the Department of Health is pumping money into services, which are expanding rapidly and provide opportunities for a variety of different kinds of working.

Child and adolescent psychiatrists nearly always work in multidisciplinary teams (with clinical psychology, social work, psychotherapy and nursing colleagues)—the varied presentation of children and families and the multiplicity of factors leading to problems making this approach essential. The doctor is not always the leader of the team: a willingness to work with others and recognize the expertise of colleagues is an essential characteristic of the successful child and adolescent psychiatrist.

Treatments in child mental health services are still predominantly psychological. The psychiatrist in the team needs basic skills in a range of psychological treatments (individual psychodynamic, cognitive/behavioural, family/systemic, etc.) and preferably a higher level of skill in one of these modalities. One of the attractions of this field for many psychiatrists is that the consultant, either alone or with colleagues, still spends a significant amount of time working directly with children. In addition, the psychiatrist must also have the necessary diagnostic skills to identify serious mental and physical illness when it presents and ensure that appropriate investigations and treatment are implemented. The biological, medical and psychological aspects of training mean that the psychiatrist has a unique contribution to the team in these areas.

Most consultants will work in multidisciplinary teams with responsibility for a defined geographical catchment area. To deal with emotional and behavioural problems in children they need to become involved with their families, their schools and the neighbourhoods in which they grow up; as a result they are often out and about in the community. A strong emphasis also placed on liaison with other services and agencies (local paediatric teams, social services, education departments, etc.) and about one third of clinical work is likely to be consultation with other staff working with children.

Models of causation are complex and multifactorial, embracing social, psychological and biological factors. Research findings are expanding exponentially and rapidly increasing our knowledge of causation, treatment and prognosis. Assessment of the child, the parents, the family, and the social environment is a time consuming but fascinating process. New assessments often take one or more one-hour sessions, meaning that you get to know children and their families as individuals. However, this also means that the work can be emotionally very stressful, especially when dealing with child abuse and its aftermath.

You need to have good communication skills and an ability to engage all family members in treatment. Persuading parents that they may have to do things differently in order to help their child whilst at the same time not making them feel blamed is a considerable skill. Many problems are not easily soluble and the capacity to live with a certain amount of uncertainty is also needed.

Within child and adolescent psychiatry there are many opportunities for subspecialism. Most consultants develop a special interest in a particular aspect of the field, for example, children with learning disabilities or chronic illness, children who have experienced abuse, or the delivery of specialist treatment such as cognitive behavioural therapy. In larger centres there will be opportunities to work full time in these areas or to work in more specialist settings such as day or inpatient units. Another option is academic child and adolescent psychiatry, which has expanded significantly in the last 15 years with most regional centres having an academic department.

Myth	Woolly minded, would-be paediatricians who never grew up.
Reality	Skilled communicators and therapists working at the cutting edge of medical, psychological and social care.
Personality	Communication and teamwork skills essential plus the capacity to cope with emotionally traumatic situations and with uncertainty.
Best aspects	Direct work with patients; varied and stimulating work life.
Worst aspects	Lack of resources (though this is improving) and living with the knowledge that you could help children but their parents won't co-operate
Requirements	MRCPsych; some paediatric experience an advantage

Hours

Junior   Consultant

Numbers 470 posts   43% are women

Competitiveness

Stress

On-calls

Junior   Consultant

Salary

£55 000   £70 000   £100 000

For further information	**Royal College of Psychiatrists** 17 Belgrave Square London SW1X 8PG Tel: 020 7235 2351 Fax: 020 7245 1231 Website: www.rcpsych.ac.uk

Old-age psychiatry

The speciality of old-age psychiatry delivers mental health services to older adults, generally aged 65 years and over. Its importance is underlined by the high levels of psychiatric morbidity in this expanding population. It exists as a separate speciality because older adults present psychiatric illness differently, have different social and family networks and have more physical illness. Conditions such as dementia, delirium and depression are commonly encountered, with new treatments for these bringing more appeal to the speciality. The considerable degree of physical and psychiatric co-morbidity brings dilemmas of diagnosis and management, and ethical issues are frequently encountered.

Old-age psychiatry services are comprehensive, covering the mental health needs of all older adults in the area. They are generally provided separately from other psychiatric services, with dedicated professionals who have received appropriate training. Services tend to be community focused and the speciality offers the opportunity for practice in a wide variety of settings, including patient's homes, residential and nursing homes, day hospitals and day centres, clinics and general and psychiatric wards. Multidisciplinary working is the norm and there is a requirement for communication between different professionals and agencies, since there is often a complex mix of psychiatric, physical and social care needs. Increasingly, links are being forged with other care providers such as social services and voluntary agencies. Services are continually developing and traditional service models are being challenged.

The workload is generally dictated by the size of the sector; the Royal College of Psychiatrists suggests a sector size of no more than 10 000 older adults per full-time consultant to result in a manageable timetable. On-call commitments vary depending on local factors; the on-call may be shared with psychiatric colleagues in other specialities but several places have a separate old-age psychiatry consultant rota. The availability of middle-grade cover is also varied, tending to be related to the number of higher trainees and staff-grade doctors. Most posts are supported by a junior trainee.

There is a great deal of academic potential in the speciality. Old-age psychiatry is increasingly represented in universities, and academic posts will usually require the possession of a higher degree. These posts may be more specialized, perhaps dedicated to dementia services, for example. Research is published in mainstream medical journals and the several journals dedicated to the speciality. Opportunities for funding of research projects are more available than previously, with support from statutory and charitable agencies. The Royal College of Psychiatrists has a Faculty of Old Age Psychiatry, which promotes academic and service developments in the speciality.

Vacancies at consultant and staff-grade level are usually available, with opportunities for part-time working and job shares. Remuneration varies, with the potential for negotiation in areas where recruitment is difficult, and the domiciliary consultation fee can increase the salary further. Opportunities for private practice are limited. The travelling involved in old-age psychiatry can be considerable and lease cars are usually available if required.

Higher training in old-age psychiatry occurs after basic psychiatric training and success in the MRCPsych examination. A specialist registrar in old-age psychiatry would undertake two years with a trainer in old-age psychiatry and a further year with a trainer in adult psychiatry or one of its subspecialities (rehabilitation, liaison or addictions) to receive a CCST in old-age psychiatry. Several higher trainees take the option of extending their training by a further year of adult psychiatry, which results in a dual CCST in old-age and adult psychiatry, particularly helpful when providing cover or on-call support for colleagues in adult psychiatry.

Myth	Old-age psychiatrists spend all their time putting confused, incontinent, old people in residential homes. Anosmia is a positive attribute to those contemplating the speciality.
Reality	A wide range of mental illness managed in the community, with an emphasis on team and inter-agency working requiring good communication and interpersonal skills. Demographic changes will result in an increasing workload and workforce.
Personality	The ability to empathize across generations is essential.
Best aspects	Varied patients and clinical settings, with holistic patient management by integrated physical, psychological and social care packages.
Worst aspects	Can be stressful, with little peer support in smaller centres.
Requirements	MRCPsych
Hours	Junior Consultant
Numbers	440 posts 27% are women
Competitiveness	
Stress	
On-calls	Junior Consultant
Salary	£min £55 000 £av £60 000 £max £85 000
For further information	**Royal College of Psychiatrists** 17 Belgrave Square London SW1X 8PG Tel: 020 7235 2351 Fax: 020 7245 1231 Website: www.rcpsych.ac.uk

The psychiatry of learning disability (mental handicap)

This speciality of psychiatry has, over the last few years, become one of the most progressive and exciting branches of psychiatry. In most parts of the country the old long-stay hospitals have closed and multidisciplinary community-based specialist health teams have developed to help in the support of people with learning disabilities living in a range of community-based settings. It is in such community and multidisciplinary settings that psychiatrists training in this speciality will work.

This term 'learning disability' has replaced that of 'mental handicap' to refer to a group of people who have a history of a significant developmental disability that has affected, to varying degrees, their intellectual and emotional development and has resulted in the presence of significant limitations in living and social and communication skills both in childhood and adult life. People with learning disabilities have high rates of emotional, psychiatric, and behaviour problems, often for very complex reasons. Psychiatrists, along with other health professionals, have the responsibility of understanding how biological, social and psychological factors may combine to give rise to the development of severe psychiatric disorders and/or the onset of serious maladaptive behaviours.

Perhaps more than in any other branch of psychiatry there is a need for a broad perspective that can encompass both an understanding of the influence of genetic and other biologically determined factors on brain development and an understanding of the influence of factors as diverse as stigma, family and carer dynamics and the person's ability to communicate his/her thoughts and feelings, on development and on the propensity to emotional and psychiatric disorders or to the onset of maladaptive behaviours. This work also challenges us ethically and legally in balancing the rights of people to make decisions about their lives against the responsibility to provide support and care for people who may not be able to make such decisions for themselves and may be at risk of abuse and exploitation.

The same challenges that are present in clinical work are also present for those engaged in research. Integration of, and collaboration between, very diverse academic disciplines is required. Those training can, for example, link to genetic research and study the relationship between specific genetically determined syndromes and particular patterns of cognitive, emotional and social development. In contrast, much research has been applied and has looked at service models and psychological treatment strategies. When it comes to research into psychiatric disorder and maladaptive behaviours affecting people with learning disabilities, there is an increasing recognition of the importance of developing models of understanding that encompass a range of perspectives from the biological to the sociological.

This speciality of psychiatry draws on diverse perspectives in a unique and demanding way. The challenge for those psychiatrists who choose to work and research in this field is to be able to integrate the advances in these diverse areas of study into both clinical practice and the development of research ideas. This branch of psychiatry has now moved out of the shadows and has in many ways leaped ahead in its thinking and in social and clinical developments. It is a privilege to work in this field, which has been for so long neglected and ignored. The time has come for the psychiatry of learning disability.

Myth	'Carers', trying to make the best of a bad job.
Reality	Busy, emotionally intense profession with medical and legal responsibilities based on scientific principle. The ability to work in a team and to manage difficult patients over a long period makes this a demanding specialty.
Personality	Broad-minded, understanding, thick-skinned. Excellent communication skills.
Best aspects	Clinical variety: no two patients are the same. Can be very emotionally rewarding. Ability to integrate a wide variety of areas into one's clinical practice
Worst aspects	Emotionally and psychologically draining a lot of the time. It is never easy. Lack of resources is a constant problem.
Requirements	MRCPsych

Hours

Junior   Consultant

Numbers 220 posts   30% are women

Competitiveness

Stress

On-calls

Junior   Consultant

Salary

£55 000   £60 000   £85 000

For further information

Royal College of Psychiatrists
17 Belgrave Square
London SW1X 8PG
Tel: 020 7235 2351
Fax: 020 7245 1231
Website: www.rcpsych.ac.uk

Psychotherapy

If you are interested in what makes people tick then psychotherapy is the career for you. Psycho-analytic psychotherapy is essentially the study of intimate relationships. It uses the relationship between the therapist and the patient as the vehicle of the therapeutic change. It is above all else a human encounter, 'being with' rather than 'doing to'. Working so closely with people, observing them develop often out of the most appalling circumstances, is an extraordinarily moving experience.

People come with a whole range of human difficulties: mental illness, physical illness, neglect, abuse, trauma. Yet, beyond the presenting complaints are fundamental problems in relating to the self and others. These can be traced back to their earliest experiences in the family. These ways of relating are recapitulated in the therapeutic relationship, which is then used as a safe place for exploration and understanding, while linking past traumatic experiences with present sympto-matology. If all goes well this enables the patient to find new and more satisfying relationships thus freeing themselves from the failures of the past. Finding and making these links is like being part of an unfolding drama which you and the patient put to rights as you go along, using the psycho-analytic model as a frame of reference. Thus, no two therapies are ever alike. This is what makes being a psychotherapist endlessly fascinating.

Therapy can be of any duration from a single meeting to several years—commonly weekly for four to 12 months. It is practised individually or in couples, families or groups. You don't have to be medically qualified to be a psychotherapist. Within the NHS a psychological therapies department will have doctors, nurses, psychologists, occupational and other therapists all trained in one or more therapeutic models. Those who don't come from these professions work predominantly in private practice. NHS consultants tend to be trained in psychoanalytic psychotherapy although some are now being trained in cognitive behaviour therapy.

In addition to NHS training most practitioners will also embark on training with one of the private psychotherapy training institutes. These trainings involve an intense study of either individ-ual or group therapy.

An essential aspect of any training is personal therapy. We all have unresolved conflicts and painful memories, which hinder our emotional and psychological development. It is therefore very important that we know as much about ourselves, our strengths and our weaknesses as possible, in order not to impose our solutions on our patients. It is also important to have an idea of what it is like to be in therapy, to understand what sort of effect what you say might have. It is, above all, an awe-inspiring and humbling experience.

The demand for psychological therapies is growing rapidly. Many are dissatisfied with traditional medicine, and analytical psychotherapy increasingly offers insight into unexplained or partially treatable medical symptoms. Yet, for the moment, medicine largely treats such patients inadequately (labelling them as 'supratentorial') and ignores psychological treatments. The future may be differ-ent and the psychotherapist may come to occupy the foreground of psychosomatic medicine.

What qualities do you need to have? Curiosity towards the human mind (including your own), thoughtfulness, patience, ability to tolerate frustration, being relatively well adjusted (ordinarily neurotic) and, perhaps above all, the capacity to enjoy life.

Myth	Middle-aged, middle-European men talking to young, attractive, articulate women about their sexual fantasies.
Reality	There are no stereotypes. A long training requiring unbounded dedication and self-motivation. Always interesting, demanding, frustrating and satisfying by turns.
Personality	Well balanced; 'must be able to think under fire' as Bion, the famous British psychoanalyst, once put it (and he was a World War I tank commander).
Best aspects	What could be more interesting than talking to people about life? It is uplifting to encounter hopefulness and courage in adversity. Continues to remain fascinating until the end of your career.
Worst aspects	Emotionally and psychologically draining a lot of the time. It is as never easy as it sounds.
Requirements	MRCPsych if pursued from the medical route

Hours

Junior · Consultant

Numbers 170

Competitiveness

Stress

On-calls

Junior · Consultant

Salary

£55 000 · £60 000 · £85 000

For further information	**Royal College of Psychiatrists** 17 Belgrave Square London SW1X 8PG Tel: 020 7235 2351 Fax: 020 7245 1231 Website: www.rcpsych.ac.uk

Forensic psychiatry

Attempting to understand the human mind and offering successful treatment to mentally troubled patients is fascinating, stressful and rewarding. This is particularly true in forensic psychiatry, the subspeciality of medicine where psychiatry and the law overlap.

Forensic psychiatrists' patients are mostly mentally disordered offenders or non-offenders with behavioural disorders. Exploring the mental states of often violent individuals is stressful, interesting and challenging and it is necessary to understand the patient as fully as possible both to plan treatment and to prognosticate, which usually includes predicting risk to others. Forensic psychiatry is unusual in that one must balance the welfare of the individual patient with the welfare of others. Forensic psychiatric patients often have multiple problems with co-existing mental illness, personality difficulties and substance abuse, making teamwork with clinical colleagues of other disciplines essential.

Most forensic psychiatrists are based in medium-security units (some in the private sector) were security depends on double-locked doors, high fences and nursing supervision in a structured and safe environment with clear psychological boundaries. Patients often spend about two years in such units. Other forensic psychiatrists work in high-security hospitals (e.g. Broadmoor) where security levels are greater and the average stay of patients is nearly eight years. Having long-stay patients allows complex understandings. Forensic psychiatrists are also frequent visitors to prisons. Apart from their inpatient work, forensic psychiatrists assess and supervise outpatients and are often called upon to give evidence in court where facing examination and cross-examination regarding such issues as psychiatric diagnosis, personality, criminal responsibility and risk leaves little place for the vagaries often associated with psychiatry. One needs to have a clear opinion of a patient, express it concisely and effectively and be willing to defend it strongly. Working with a wide multi-agency group including the police, Home Office and lawyers is often interesting and challenging. A knowledge of relevant legislation is essential and a lot of paperwork is generated.

Specialist registrar training in forensic psychiatry is well structured nationally and covers all relevant aspects of practice. Specialist registrars rarely have difficulty in obtaining a consultant job quickly and on good terms.

Forensic psychiatry is an expanding speciality with a youthful exuberance, often modern working environments and scope for personal professional development. Academic posts in forensic psychiatry are growing and academic potential is good. Superspecialization is also emerging, such as forensic psychotherapy and forensic child and adolescent psychiatry.

Good forensic psychiatrists are usually curious, decisive and opinionated and although they choose to care for society's unloved and unwanted they remain realistic. They are often obsessional and thrive on analysing and overcoming complexity. An ability insightfully to understand others and environments is important. Coping with anxieties, usually relating to risk, and holding anxieties for others is part of the work. The patients are often of a high profile and if they reoffend one needs to cope with the subsequent inquiry and defend one's actions. Effectively separating professional and personal life is vital: stepping into the mind of someone who has killed may be fascinating, but one must never forget to step out again at the end of the interview! One should not practise forensic psychiatry for gratitude from patients or the public as presents are infrequent. It is a subspeciality that provides rewards in other ways.

Myth	A medical Sherlock Holmes caring for Hannibal Lecter.
Reality	Fascinating work on the margin of medicine and the law, involving patients on the margin of society who have often gone beyond the law.
Personality	Rather obsessional realists who can overcome challenge, thrive on complexity and cope with anxiety
Best aspects	Time to explore and understand the darker recesses of the human mind whilst working in varied settings with interesting colleagues from many different disciplines and agencies. Good and varied professional development potential.
Worst aspects	Patients who can seriously harm others, resulting in distress and inquiries into your work. A lot of paperwork
Requirements	MRCPsych

Hours

Junior — Consultant

Numbers 150 consultants; 76 specialist registrars

Competitiveness

Stress

On-calls

Junior — Consultant

Salary

£75 000 — £105 000 — £140 000

For further information	**Royal College of Psychiatrists** 17 Belgrave Square London SW1X 8PG Tel: 020 7235 2351 Fax: 020 7245 1231 Website: www.rcpsych.ac.uk

CHAPTER 11
The Armed Forces

The Army

'Why did you join the Army?' remains a very common question and parallels the very classic medical school interview question 'Why do you want to be a doctor?' Some people have a very snappy answer but in most cases the answer comprises a rather ill-defined combination of factors. Many have enjoyed their involvement with the officer training corps at university and realize there is an additional dimension to life in the Army beyond practising medicine within the NHS. It's worth noting that a military cadetship offers a very comfortable existence as a clinical student and few will regret the decision to join.

As a cadet in the Royal Army Medical Corps you can expect a comfortable salary far in excess of the student grant. You will meet other cadets from around the country and you will have the opportunity to apply for a student elective in a military hospital overseas or where there are military contacts. For example, military cadets have recently completed electives in trauma centres in the USA and Australia. Once qualified, you will do your preregistration year in military units or, if you prefer, in NHS hospitals. You may then apply, if desired, to do an SHO job (accident and emergency is a popular choice) before starting the entry officer's (EO) course at Sandhurst at the Defence Medical Services Training Centre. These four months prepare you to be a regimental medical officer and include physical and leadership training plus education in military medicine, tropical medicine and military surgery. Every officer will do, and is expected to pass, an advanced life support course and a battlefield advanced trauma life support course (officially recognized equivalent of the advanced trauma life support course, or ATLS).

As a regimental medical officer you may be posted to a prestigious ceremonial unit, or train for your 'wings' with an airborne unit or be involved as medical support on peace-keeping and peace-enforcement missions around the world. Where you will be is very much determined by the interests and abilities you display on the EO course. But wherever you are you will be responsible not only for the primary care of soldiers and their families, but also for the training of your combat medics and for providing emergency medical support for your unit on exercise and on operations. There are many opportunities in the Army to develop traditional sporting interests and to further your professional development.

The Army supports its officers in attending the necessary modular training courses for their specialties and encourages them to be involved in teaching, research and the publication of articles and books. It would be naïve to fail to recognize the recent changes in the Defence Medical Services; in particular there has been a reduction in the number of Service hospitals both in the UK and abroad. However, what has replaced these are three 'Ministry of Defence Hospital Units' (MDHUs) within the NHS district general hospitals. These are integrated units where military, medical and nursing staff work alongside their civilian counterparts. The MDHUs are in Camberley, Plymouth, Northallerton, Cosham (?2005) and Peterborough and, in theory, will offer greater training possibilities in the acute specialties than the previous small military hospitals. Every 'teeth arm' (infantry and tanks) unit will still require a regimental medical officer and the primary care role of the doctor in the Army remains firmly established.

Myth	Can't get a job anywhere else.
Reality	Breeds strong character; works in diverse and challenging environments; strong support to develop postgraduate training in chosen career pathway.
Best aspects	Sponsorship as student; travel, sport, opportunities outside mainstream medicine; postgraduate training including overseas attachment. No need to look for another job for six years. Generous non-contributory pension scheme.
Worst aspects	Uncertainty of posting; worries (usually unfounded) about NHS employment on leaving; no way out for six years.
Requirements	Undergraduates (Cadetship scheme for final three years); UK registration (direct entrants)

Hours

Junior
(always on duty when singlehanded)

Consultant

Numbers	cadets: 100 doctors: 400

Competitiveness

Stress

On-calls

Junior

Consultant
(dependent on specialty)

Salary	£11–13 000 (student) £25 500 (house officer) £42 000 (end of six years) £50–80 000 (senior officer/consultant)
For further information	**Officer Recruiting** RHQ Royal Army Medical Corps Keogh Barracks Ash Vale Aldershot GU12 5RQ Tel: 01252 340309 Fax: 01252 340224 E-mail: rhq.ramc@clara.net Website: http://www.army.mod.uk

The Royal Air Force

The medical branch of the Royal Air Force (RAF) offers opportunities in general practice, in a number of hospital-based specialties and in medical administration. There are unique appointments in aviation and occupational medicine. General duties medical officers receive considerable training and experience in aviation and occupational medicine and all medical officers are likely to spend some time on flying stations. Patients include all RAF personnel, their dependants in some circumstances, personnel from the other Armed Services and NATO and (for hospital doctors) NHS patients.

Entry is by a short service commission (SSC) of six years, although fully trained medical officers can ask for a SSC of three years. Medical students make use of the bursary and cadetship schemes allowing for sponsorship throughout medical undergraduate studies. Cadets receive RAF pay, allowances and tuition fees and have opportunities to visit RAF units at home and abroad. All cadets are given the opportunity to learn to fly with the University Air Squadrons. One or both preregistration house jobs may be done in a Service hospital and on full registration as a Flight Lieutenant, you complete six further years in uniform. Initial general training is followed by a posting to an RAF station. Full training for general practice is available in approved appointments. Those planning a career in a hospital specialty are offered general professional/basic specialist training; acquisition of the appropriate diploma should allow progression to higher training as a specialist registrar. However, completion of specialist registrar training to CCST would require extension of the engagement, usually by taking a permanent commission (PC). Hospital specialties include general medicine, surgery, orthopaedics, anaesthetics, ENT, ophthalmology, pathology, radiology, rheumatology, rehabilitation and psychiatry. There are occasional opportunities in other specialties.

Qualified doctors below the age of 39 years on entry may apply to join the RAF on SSCs and will follow training programmes depending on their own and the Services' needs. Fully trained practitioners, either GPs or hospital consultants, may also enter on SSCs.

A medical officer with an SSC may apply at any stage for a permanent commission, but this is usually after two years. This entails a commitment to serve for at least 16 years and allows completion of training (if required) and some years of practice as a GP principal or hospital consultant. Those wishing to train in occupational or public health medicine are selected from those already holding PCs.

Professional life in the RAF medical branch is satisfying but somewhat unpredictable, being greatly influenced by factors such as international emergencies and changes in the greater RAF. Recently, a series of Defence reviews has caused exceptional turbulence. Although the dust is now settling, further changes must be expected in terms and conditions of service when the implications of the Bett report become clear.

Whatever the future holds, the RAF needs its uniformed medical branch, continues to make a massive investment in training at all levels and provides a setting for medical practice of the highest standard. Factors appreciated by RAF medical officers include the *esprit de corps*, the family atmosphere and privileges of an officers' mess, the excellent sporting facilities, the company of a highly trained and qualified body of professionals and tradesmen in other callings, a good life for families, but especially the chance to practise their chosen specialty among a highly discriminating and well-informed clientele.

Myth	Light-blue mountebanks with beer foam on their handlebar moustaches.
Reality	Wide variety, common thread, a taste for the unusual, the demanding and the exciting; interest in aviation and technology helpful.
Personality	Extrovert sociable optimists (10% grumbling time allowance).
Best aspects	Training, quality of practice, company and social life, travel, organization, morale, sporting facilities, adventure.
Worst aspects	Restricted choices, unpopular postings, family separations.
Requirements	University (bursary, cadetship) UK registration (direct entrants).

Hours

Junior   Consultant

Numbers — 240 posts   approximately 20% are women (no restriction on numbers)

Competitiveness

Stress

On-calls

Junior   Consultant

Salary — ±11–13 000 (student); £25 500 (house officer); £42 000 (end of six years); £50–80 000 (senior officer/consultant)

For further information

Medical Liaison Officer
Directorate of Recruiting, Selection (Royal Air Force)
PO Box 1000
Cranwell
Sleaford
Lincolnshire NG34 8GZ
Tel: 01400 261201 (ext. 6811)
E-mail: mdlo@raf.net
Website: www.raf-careers.com

The Royal Navy

From day one in the Royal Navy, medical officers will find themselves not only as doctors and leaders of a medical team, but also as officers integrated into the wider activities of the workplace be that of a ship, submarine, shore base or commando unit.

You may join for your final three years at medical school on a cadetship, subject to passing the Admiralty Interview Board. The 'return of service' (ROS) (pay-back in order words) is the whole of the six-year SCC staring after the preregistration house officer year. Thus the maximum initial relationship with the Royal Navy is 10 years. Qualified doctors may join at any time subject to the same selection process. Students are paid £33 000 over three years made up of salary and grant (1999/2000 rates); even tuition fees are paid for you. Withdrawal is allowed up to the award of your degree (with a financial penalty).

The SCC satrts with a four-month course to prepare you for your role in the Royal Navy: eight weeks at the Britannia Royal Naval College is followed by courses in occupational, aviation and diving medicine, management of clinical problems at sea and combat casualty care to mention but a few.

The next two and a half years are spent providing primary care in a 'general duties' setting. The varied range includes gaining the coveted Royal Marine green beret and serving with 3 Commando Brigade Royal Marines in the Arctic, jungle and desert; or going to sea on one of HM frigates to the West Indies, Falklands, Gulf or Far East; or with HMS *Endurance* for six months in the Antarctic. As well as being the doctor for all on board you may become ship's diver, 'bridge watch-keeper' or sports and entertainment officer. At sea you are likely to be winched from a helicopter to another ship to treat a casualty, or be tasked to provide humanitarian aid to a civilian community. As a submariner you play a vital role as part of Britain's nuclear deterrent.

The next three years of your SCC are devoted to basic specialist or general practice vocational training. Opportunities exist in all the major disciplines except paediatrics, obstetrics and gynaecology. Training is governed by the Royal Colleges as it is for our NHS colleagues and most will complete general practice vocational training or gain their basic higher professional exam during this period. For those opting for a longer commission, the Services grant as many specialist registrar training numbers as they require to suitable candidates, crucially avoiding the dire rat race for aspiring NHS trainees; our training rotations are second to none.

The main attraction of an SCC, or at least as important as the financial sponsorship, is the opportunity to travel and for three years to experience the sort of life that NHS SHOs and general practice vocational trainees can only dream of while staying in touch with medicine. Apart from a very different general duties job, diving, skiing, mountaineering and trans-ocean sailing all figure regularly, helped by your friendly commanding officer! So if you're not in a rush to become a consultant but want to be assured of excellent training after three years and to develop your leadership skills as well as the variety of different activities then an SCC in the Royal Navy Medical Service might well suit you. Why not find out and visit us at our expense?

Myth	Play a lot of golf, run the mess bar.
Reality	Opportunity to combine medicine with travel, adventure and challenge together with postgraduate training opportunities after three years that are second to none.
Personality	Leadership, independent thinker, cool under pressure, flexible, team player.
Best aspects	Sponsorship as student; travel, sport, excitement and 'life' experiences outside mainstream medicine, generous non-contributory pension scheme, six weeks' holiday a year; no requirement to look for the next job for six years.
Worst aspects	At beck and call of the director of medical officer appointments, two to three years' general duties with little opportunity for formal postgraduate training during that time; worries about employment in the NHS on completion of commission; committed to six years after full registration.
Requirements	Satisfactory completion of year 2 at medical school (cadet); provisional or full registration (direct entry).

Hours

Junior [always on duty when single handed]   Consultant

Numbers   25 per year (mainly cadetships, some direct entries)

Competitiveness

Stress

but very variable.

On-calls

Junior   Consultant

Salary   £11–13 000 (student), £25 500 (house officer), up to £42 000 SCC (end of six years), £50–80 000 (HPT/specialist registrar)

For further information
Med. Pers. 2N
Room 133
Victory Building
HM Naval Base
Portsmouth PO1 3LS
Tel: 02392 727818
Fax: 02392 727805
Website: www.royal-navy.mod.uk/rnmedical/

CHAPTER 12

Pathology

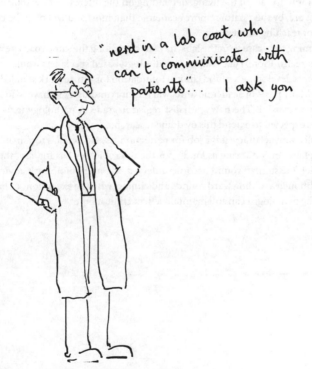

"nerd in a lab coat who can't communicate with patients"... I ask you

Overview

The classical image of the harried pathologist up to his elbows in a post mortem or of the immunologist excitedly watching DNA crawl across an electrophoretic strip does not represent the whole truth in these fields. The worlds of the laboratory and mortuary are not as wholly separated from clinical medicine as many physicians would suggest. We all rely on laboratory services for all our blood tests and it is them we call for advice on what to do with the results. It goes without saying that they are assumed to be accurate. Post-mortems, frozen sections and routine cytology are likewise taken for granted.

All the pathological/laboratory services have some degree of clinical input, some more than others. Haematology is invariably both a clinical and laboratory-based service whilst histopathology can have a minimal input to care of the living, depending on the interests of the individual concerned. All the specialties are, by their nature, more academic than most and will often be combined with a strong research or teaching interest.

All trainees aiming for a career 'in the labs' have to start along the same road as everyone else, but only as far as full registration. That said, most pathology-based specialists would agree that spending one or two years developing a sound clinical foundation for future work should be considered as time well spent. Many posts in academic units will require candidates to have MRCP in addition to MRCPath, to be successful. The new specialist registrar grade in pathology takes four years, but most trainees are expected to extend this by doing research.

Pathology is all about accuracy: it is a job for perfectionists. No detail is too small, no minutia too minute. The applause may not ring as loudly for the microbiologist as for, say, the cardiothoracic surgeon, but when the sternal wound becomes infected, the microbiologist's advice will be sought soon enough. Although avoiding ward rounds and clinics (with the exceptions of haematology and immunology), the pathologist can still maintain a firm clinical input.

Pathology: career pathway

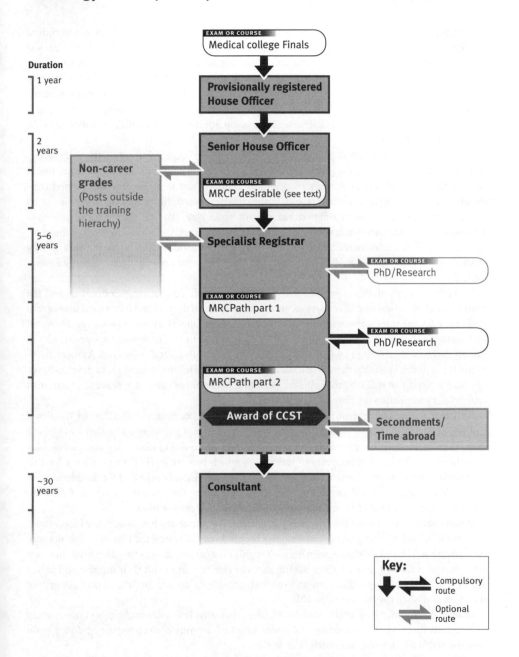

EXAM OR COURSE
Medical college Finals

Duration

1 year

Provisionally registered House Officer

2 years

Senior House Officer

EXAM OR COURSE
MRCP desirable (see text)

Non-career grades
(Posts outside the training hierachy)

5–6 years

Specialist Registrar

EXAM OR COURSE
PhD/Research

EXAM OR COURSE
MRCPath part 1

EXAM OR COURSE
PhD/Research

EXAM OR COURSE
MRCPath part 2

Award of CCST

Secondments/ Time abroad

~30 years

Consultant

Key:

Compulsory route

Optional route

Chemical pathology

Chemical pathologists provide an important link between clinical chemistry laboratories and clinical medicine. Consequently, chemical pathologists must have an extensive knowledge of both clinical chemistry and medicine. As formal training is mainly in laboratory medicine, it is becoming increasingly important that the individual has a good grounding in clinical medicine before starting Higher Specialist Training (HST). The CCST in chemical pathology is obtained on gaining membership to the Royal College of Pathologists and on completing satisfactory training. Membership is normally obtained by passing the College's examination but it might be considered following submission of published works.

What makes chemical pathology such an interesting and challenging specialty is the wide variety of tasks undertaken. One of the principal functions is to advise clinicians on the optimum use of clinical chemistry laboratory services to diagnose, monitor and treat diseases and related conditions, and on the interpretation of results. Approximately two thirds of consultants are involved in direct patient management often running joint endocrine, diabetic or metabolic clinics—subspecialties of medicine that involve significant laboratory input. Others are involved in the management of patients in intensive care units or on parenteral nutrition. There is also the opportunity to specialize, for example in paediatric clinical chemistry and in the investigation of inherited metabolic disorders.

In addition to the clinical component there is the scientific or analytical component and the management of a diagnostic laboratory service for both hospital doctors and GPs. Good managerial skills are essential as the consultant works closely with other laboratory professionals and hospital staff in the development of services and the allocation of resources. There is ample opportunity to undertake research, either on one's own or in collaboration with clinical colleagues. As there are so many facets to this specialty, there is considerable opportunity for the incumbent to develop his or her own interest and skills, be they clinical, scientific academic or computer-related, constrained only by resources within the hospital or institution.

Although not a requirement, a trainee should consider obtaining membership of the Royal College of Physicians before embarking on a career in chemical pathology. The Part I MRCPath examination—two written examination papers covering all aspects of laboratory and clinical biochemistry—is taken after three years of training of which two are in HST. In preparing for this examination, many trainees obtain an MSc in clinical biochemistry. For the Part II examination, the trainee has to undertake a dissertation, with some developing their research interests further in order to obtain an MD or PhD, and to pass a practical and oral examination.

When considering a career as a chemical pathologist, it is important to visit as many laboratories as possible in both district general and teaching hospitals and to review the role of a consultant in each situation. The trainee should then decide roughly on a career pathway based on his or her own interests and skills and seek a trainee post in departments that most suit their interest and career aspirations. Additional qualifications and research experience do improve the chances of getting the plum jobs when they become available.

Chemical pathology is an exciting and rewarding specialty. It is a demanding job testing many different attributes of the individual. For those who feel nervous at the prospect of doing brain surgery, chemical pathology is a much safer option.

Myth	A doctor who prefers spending most of the time on the telephone, playing with computers or fiddling under the bonnet of a large analyser.
Reality	A challenging and rewarding subspecialty of pathology that involves a training in both medicine and biochemistry, providing excellent opportunities for clinical patient management, research and teaching.
Personality	Must be a good communicator and a diplomat and have good managerial skills.
Best aspects	A combination of science and medicine. It is rewarding making a diagnosis on a minimum data set while the clinician waits for the results of complex, often irrelevant, investigations.
Worst aspects	Dealing with stubborn, demanding clinicians who refuse to see reason or common sense when approached about the inappropriateness of out-of-hours investigations.
Requirements	MRCPath and MRCP or MD/PhD beneficial

Hours

Junior   Consultant

Numbers	218 posts (seven per year) 10% are women

Competitiveness

Stress

On-calls

Junior   Consultant

Salary

£56 000   £65 000   £100 000

For further information	**Royal College of Pathologists** 2 Carlton House Terrace London SW1Y 5AF Tel: 020 7930 5861 Fax: 020 7321 0523 Website: www.rcpath.org

Forensic pathology

Forensic medicine can be considered as medical disciplines that assist the law and the administration of justice. Under this umbrella may be considered such specialties as forensic pathology, forensic psychiatry and clinical forensic medicine. If a wider definition is being used, a medically qualified lawyer, a coroner or advisor to a medical defence organization could also be included.

Forensic pathology is one of the divisions of pathology. The specialty is not just the examination of victims of murder, but the examination of all aspects of death where there are medicolegal implications. The casework must then be prepared and presented in a legal forum. Forensic pathology has an important role in public health. Many forensic pathologists review clinical cases of assault. The investigation of war crimes and other abuses of human rights has been an increasing role for forensic medicine. As well as performing autopsies, forensic pathologists have significant teaching and research duties, especially the university-based pathologists. Forensic pathologists need to work as part of a team, which is not just medical, but will include the coroner, police, forensic scientists and lawyers, as well as running a laboratory. Good communication skills are vital. It has often been said (by those who do not know pathology), that doctors with poor communication skills are ideally suited to pathology. This is particularly untrue with all forensic disciplines where you are only as good as the evidence you give and the way you give it.

Trainees have to undergo an initial period of training in histopathology and may then complete their training in forensic pathology. Membership of the Royal College of Pathologists may be taken on forensic pathology or histopathology but if the latter training and exam are completed, a recognized diploma in forensic pathology will be required. Two are currently available: the Diploma in Forensic Pathology of the Royal College of Pathologists and the Diploma in Medical Jurisprudence (pathology) offered by the Worshipful Society of Apothecaries. The advantage of completing training in histopathology is that it allows one to obtain a consultant post in histopathology, whilst having membership in forensic pathology limits you to forensic pathology. This would not matter if there were large numbers of departments of forensic pathology, but there are not.

Full-time positions in forensic pathology have traditionally been university based. However, in England and Wales there are now only units in London (at Guys and St George's), Cardiff, and Sheffield. Liverpool and Newcastle currently have a single senior post each, and only Sheffield has an established Chair. The situation in Scotland is better, with departments in Aberdeen, Dundee, Edinburgh and Glasgow, the latter three departments having a Chair. There is also a State Department in Northern Ireland, with links with Queen's University. As well as full-time posts, consultant histopathologists with training in forensic pathology act as Home Office Pathologists, and there are a number of independent practitioners. In England and Wales, once training is complete, accreditation by the Home Office is required. There are fewer than 50 practitioners on the list. The structure and funding of forensic pathology in England and Wales may be reviewed in the future.

Most practitioners of clinical forensic medicine, often called forensic physicians or police surgeons, are GPs with some extra training. Many take the Diploma in Medical Jurisprudence (clinical). They are contracted to work directly for the police. Some police forces have block contracts with companies to provide clinical forensic services, which include the examination of living victims of assault and people in custody.

Myth	Television doctor who stands in a muddy field staring at a mutilated corpse and eating a sandwich.
Reality	Doctor who stands in a muddy field staring at a mutilated corpse (sometimes).
Personality	Strong, resilient person who is a good communicator and able to work for long periods at odd hours as part of a team.
Best aspects	Interesting and varied case work. Never knowing what's next. 'Finding the answer'. Assisting in the administration of justice.
Worst aspects	Being messed around by the courts. Frequent nights without sleep on call. No decent career structure.
Requirements	MRCPath, Diploma in Forensic Pathology

Hours

Junior   Consultant

Numbers   55 posts   10% are women

Competitiveness

Stress

On-calls

Junior   Consultant

Salary

£60 000   £85 000   £150 000

For further information	**Royal College of Pathologists** 2 Carlton House Terrace London SW1Y 5AF Tel: 020 7930 5861 Fax: 020 7321 0523 Website: www.rcpath.org

Haematology

Haematology is both fascinating and fun and most junior doctors rotating through a clinical haematology post enjoy it, with many going on to make a career of it. In what other specialty can a doctor shuffle between such a range as in haematology: molecular biologist, clinical geneticist, laboratory manager, geriatrician, paediatrician, bone marrow transplanter, immunologist, protein chemist, pattern recognizer (morphology), discussion of evolutionary genetic drift, computing, budgeting, etc.? In addition one manages a unique range of haematological malignancies ('blood cancers') and diseases only found in ethnic minorities. This involves working with groups of patients with lifelong high medical need and requires particular care. There are fascinating possibilities of combining high science, such as gene therapy, with clinical care with an ease not shared by many other specialties. The opportunities for personal and academic refreshment grow ever bigger and more exciting with the development of more training and collaborations across Europe as well as the Internet and cheaper travel.

As a result of the great variety of opportunities and increased subspecialization, haematology has become the chosen specialty of a wide variety of characters from the extrovert transplanter/intensivist to the often more introverted specialist morphologist. While most haematologists are primarily clinicians with routine laboratory management roles or research roles, there remain interesting possibilities as Director of Pathology (or medicine) for consultants to develop as managers, strategists and leaders.

On-call varies during rotations in training but most junior doctors are now either resident for the clinical needs of the haematology department or available by phone to give advice on haematological disease in patients, interpretation of laboratory tests, appropriate use of blood products and transfusion problems. The local consultants are always available for back-up advice and support, as are the specialist consultants from the National Blood Transfusion Service.

Haematology has attracted a wide variety of individuals. Although, as yet, few women have been awarded professional chairs, there are a remarkably high number of women consultants and trainees compared with many hospital specialties. Above all, you need to be interested in some of the disease processes of the blood and be able to communicate with either patients or with other doctors and your laboratory staff, or your research colleagues.

Entry to haematology training follows membership to the Royal College of Physicians. It is a four-year specialist curriculum designed by the Royal College of Pathologists and is now well structured, offering experience and education in the management of bleeding diatheses and thrombophilia, paediatric and geriatric haematology and leukaemias (both acute and chronic) with high technology, routine and palliative care approaches, as well as the inherited anaemias, to name but some of the areas.

Classically, haematologists have, in addition to their specialist training, undertaken two or more years of research for an MD thesis. Their MD research can be laboratory, clinical or mixed. Increasingly opportunities to work within the Cochrane collaboration, performing systematic reviews and acquiring critical appraisal skills, are being taken up by doctors and valued by their future colleagues.

The MRCPath is taken as a specialist registrar in two parts: the first (Diploma in Pathology), after two years which involves two three-hour essay papers followed by practicals, testing, interpretation of morphology and laboratory investigations (including coagulation, transfusion and electrophoresis) and a viva. The second part is by two vivas which are general or specialist, relating to the examinee's research or areas of particular interest.

Myth	Mousy laboratory backroom boys or gung-ho transplanters.
Reality	A developing and expanding field that has developed clinical expertise of its own while remaining essential to most other hospital activities.
Personality	Varied, ranging from transplanters and intensivists to those providing continuing care to geriatric patients with grumbling blood disorders.
Best aspects	At the cutting edge of science, including molecular biology, protein chemistry and crystallography. The immediate application of results of tests performed in your own laboratory to your own patients. The ever-improving cure rate for high-grade malignancies. The community care and genetic counselling aspects of inherited diseases.
Worst aspects	Major transfusion or coagulation problems at the end of a bank holiday weekend. The perpetual rise in laboratory workload and expectations of new tests and technology allied to continued demands for budget savings.
Requirements	MRCP and MRCPath

Hours

Junior   Consultant

Numbers 595 posts 28% are women

Competitiveness

Stress

On-calls

Junior   Consultant

Salary

£min   £av   £max

£50 000   £62 000   £100 000

For further information	**Royal College of Pathologists** 2 Carlton House Terrace London SW1Y 5AF Tel: 020 7930 5861 Fax: 020 7321 0523 Website: www.rcpath.org

Transfusion medicine

Transfusion medicine, the Cinderella specialty of haematology, is finally preparing to go to the ball; anyone who goes with her will not be bored! As the public and profession become increasingly aware that blood transfusion is a complex medical intervention with specific benefits and hazards, the skills and knowledge of consultants in transfusion medicine are in demand and appreciated.

There are three distinct aspects to the discipline:

(1) The core function is the provision of sufficient, safe blood components and products and advice on their appropriate use. Obtaining suitable donors requires media skills and an understanding of the sociophysiology of donors. The subsequent testing and processing of blood require a knowledge of microbiology and interest in innovative technologies, information technology skills and teamwork. Advising on the appropriate use (which surprisingly is not well understood) brings close contact with clinicians in hospitals. The impending advent of blood substitutes and further development of all forms of blood conservation policies (e.g. blood salvage during surgery) pose new challenges.

(2) The scientific basis of red cell, white cell and platelet immunobiology and genetics has led to the development of specialist diagnostic laboratories located in transfusion centres. The clinical applications include: (for red cells) the prophylaxis and management of haemolytic disease of the newborn; (for white cells) the HLA system, which underpins all transplant work; and (for platelets) the investigation and management of all thrombocytopenias from neonatal to iatrogenic.

(3) Tissue banking including bone and skin banking is gradually coming into the regulatory environment of the blood transfusion services. Cord blood banks have been developed by transfusion specialists and are located in blood transfusion centres.

Any one of these aspects may become a subspecialty within the specialty.

Consultants in transfusion medicine as a rule do not have their own patients, hence the lack of a certain glamour in the profession, nevertheless therapeutic plasma exchange and stem cell harvesting for transplantation bring direct patient contact. There are also an increasing number of joint appointments with hospitals and academic units which provide direct responsibility for patients and wide opportunities for research.

Most consultants in transfusion medicine are haematologists but there are opportunities for microbiologists and immunologists. The regulatory environment in which the blood transfusion service works provides close contact and understanding of the workings of the European Union.

Since the subject is very broad the ability to create one's own job according to one's interest is rewarded by great job satisfaction.

Myth	Transfusion centres are simple blood dairies.
Reality	Transfusion medicine embraces a wide range of interests, most of which have an important interface with clinical medicine. A substantial number of consultants have joint appointments with clinical duties.
Personality	All personalities can be catered for from the reserved, private person to the outgoing eccentric. There are also many opportunities for doctors of other than consultant grade in the service: associate specialist/staff grade. These posts too can be very rewarding.
Best aspects	The varied nature of the work. The opportunity to develop one's interests and to contribute to the maturing of a still young discipline with international interests.
Worst aspects	Still perceived as a backwater specialty.
Requirements	MRCP and MRCPath

Hours

Junior   Consultant

Numbers   70 posts   60% are women

Competitiveness

Stress

On-calls

Junior   Consultant

Salary

£50 000   £65 000   £100 000

For further information	Royal College of Pathologists 2 Carlton House Terrace London SW1Y 5AF Tel: 020 7930 5861 Fax: 020 7321 0523 Website: www.rcpath.org

Histopathology and cytopathology

A career in histopathology starts at SHO level. During this post, there may be (new proposals) an assessment of aptitude at six to nine months. Specialist registrar posts follow, with a Part 1 written and practical examination at two and a half years and the awarding of the DipRCPath; then Part 2 at four and a half years, after which MRCPath is awarded. The training during these years is definitely hands-on: describing, cutting up and sampling surgical specimens, learning to report cytology and frozen sections, autopsy technique and research methods. Specialist registrars are based in rotations between teaching and district general hospitals and between subspecialty areas. The broad intention is to allow maximum exposure to the range of volume of material you could be called upon to report in consultant practice.

So what personal characteristics make for a good diagnostic pathologist?

- a visual (not necessarily photographic) memory helps;
- the ability to extract the essential diagnostic histological features from a large area of distracting and non-contributory elements and to interpret them in a clinical context;
- a very good grasp of how to convey that interpretation in clear written prose such that there can be no misunderstanding: the report and slides are stored forever and don't dissolve like sutures over the years.
- it helps to be reasonably good with your hands, as you are going to spend a lot of your time dissecting out the areas of tissue on which you will base your diagnoses.

So what's the job like? It is hospital-based but (unless you needle lumps and bumps yourself) without direct patient contact—there are no clinics, no ward rounds. Your office will be in a lab block and you will spend most of your day looking down a microscope scrutinizing cells (cytology) and tissues (histopathology). You will write or dictate reports; these are printed and you will then spend a lot of time proofreading them before you sign them out. You will show and discuss these cases at meetings with the various teams who sent them. Post-mortems are less of a feature than they were even 10 years ago, although many district general hospital consultants perform autopsies for the coroner, a lucrative if time-consuming sideline.

Senior lectureships are there for the research minded. In such posts it may be possible to end up doing no diagnostic service work relating directly to patients. However, most manage to juggle research and research supervision, teaching and routine diagnostic reporting. The larger centres, usually teaching hospitals, have areas of histopathology subspecialization, such as paediatric and renal pathology, or neuropathology. Even in a small district general hospital there may be some division of the work—one consultant may do the bulk of the cytology or the dermatopathology, for example—and this trend towards subspecialization is increasing.

Given appropriate consultant staffing levels, this is a stimulating, mentally challenging and highly responsible job which puts you at the hub of clinical diagnosis and patient management. When, through sickness or retirement, there are not enough consultants for the workload, it can get fairly grim, adversely affecting your social and family life. Consider that even the most mundane basal cell carcinoma is not a basal cell carcinoma until *you* report it as such. The job is no nine-to-five refuge for the ward weary. Fine, you don't have to do bloods or on-call, but you live with the knowledge that a one-letter typo ('is completely excised' instead of 'incompletely excised') can make the difference between an early curative re-excision and a later recurrence and spread. So, in summary, this job is stimulating but hardly the doss many of our colleagues think it is.

Myth	Being bleeped by grumpy nine-to-fivers when you're on a ward round to moan about details on a request form you wrote at midnight on call. Evisceration merchants.
Reality	Usually friendly nit-pickers just covering your back and looking to maximize chances of successful diagnosis for the patient.
Personality	Tough, thorough, able to reach reliable diagnostic decisions and defend them.
Best aspects	Close liaison with clinical teams, providing diagnosis and advice, ensuring optimal patient treatment.
Worst aspects	Too many clinical teams sending us work—histopathology has not kept pace with consultant expansions in other fields, although recently this may be improving.
Requirements	MRCPath, BSc helpful

Hours

Junior   Consultant

Numbers   836 posts (83 per year)   29% are women

Competitiveness

Stress

On-calls	none	none, unless specialist centre
	Junior	Consultant

Salary

£50 000   £62 000   £100 000

For further information	**Royal College of Pathologists** 2 Carlton House Terrace London SW1Y 5AF Tel: 020 7930 5861 Fax: 020 7321 0523 Website: www.rcpath.org

Immunology

Compared with most other medical specialties, clinical immunology is a young discipline. Nevertheless, it is now a very well established one, accepted as having an essential place in any comprehensive healthcare system.

At its inception, clinical immunology was largely a laboratory-based diagnostic specialty which sought to apply the knowledge and techniques of the rapidly developing field of fundamental scientific immunology to patient care. However, there has been a shift in emphasis to include a very definite element of clinical work involving hands-on patient contact. Thus, a typical consultant clinical immunologist will have responsibility not only for directing the activities of a diagnostic immunology laboratory manned by professional technical staff, but also for the running his or her own (mainly outpatient) clinical service.

Immunology laboratories generally offer a well circumscribed range of tests used in the diagnosis and monitoring of autoimmune conditions, immunodeficiencies, allergies and some blood disorders. A number of more esoteric tests are likely only to be of interest to the consultant immunologist in the management of his or her own patients. As far as clinical work is concerned, there is one defining group of patients who are looked after by an immunologist—those with primary immunodeficiencies, rare conditions which often need considerable specialist knowledge in their investigation and management. The rest of the work is a moveable feast which is very much determined by the individual's own interest and the extent of local demand for them (e.g. they may have a strong interest in allergy).

By any standards, clinical immunology is a small specialty, with very few posts outside major teaching hospitals—a situation which is unlikely to change. Unsurprisingly, therefore, the political scene tends to be dominated, at any one time, by the voices of a small number of prominent figures. Although this is not necessarily bad, it can make the discipline seem rather claustrophobic. Trainees rapidly become aware of who's who in the field and get round to meeting most of them at some point in their training. If you are thinking of a career in immunology, anyone working in the specialty will be able to tell you where to turn for advice, if they can't offer it themselves, and it's sensible to consult more than one source.

Those considering immunology as a career probably have a fairly intellectual mindset and are keen on the scientific aspects of medical practice. In addition, they need to be prepared to compete for places in a small field, both at entry level (acceptance into the specialist registrar grade after gaining the MRCP) and at exit level (appointment as a consultant after MRCPath). The pursuit of a higher degree (MD or PhD) and the production of publications are likely to be positive career moves, so an aversion to research is unhelpful. A formal training programme for clinical immunology, jointly agreed by the Royal College of Physicians and the Royal College of Pathologists, should serve to standardize and expedite training in the specialty. A minority of trainees extend their clinical repertoire in order to aim for dual accreditation in immunology *and* medicine, potentially increasing the number of career options ultimately available to them.

Although a few centres have more than one consultant, a high proportion of posts remain single-handed, so there's a fair chance that you will begin your consultant career as head of your own department, with all the managerial responsibility which that entails.

Myth	Ivory tower dwellers, specializing in an esoteric subject with limited relevance to the real world and which nobody else understands (or would want to).
Reality	A major contributor to 'routine' laboratory diagnosis. The only port of call for patients with certain conditions. Stimulating, but not necessarily 'rocket science'.
Personality	Intellectual rigour, self-reliance, ability to work in isolation but still communicate effectively with everyone else.
Best aspects	Offers great insight into the relationship between laboratory and clinical medicine. Finding the answers others haven't found. Having sole responsibility when things go well.
Worst aspects	Communication with peers is often at a distance. Having sole responsibility when things go badly.
Requirements	MRCP *and* MRCPath; MD or PhD helps

Hours

Junior   Consultant

Numbers   40 posts (five per year)

Competitiveness

Stress

On-calls

Junior   Consultant

Salary

£45 000   £55 000   £65 000

For further information

Royal College of Pathologists
2 Carlton House Terrace
London SW1Y 5AF
Tel: 020 7930 5861
Fax: 020 7321 0523
Website: www.rcpath.org

Microbiology

Microbes are the most significant life form sharing this planet with humans. One of the reasons for their successful existence is utilization of any available food source including humans whose defences may be breached. The ubiquitous presence and the astronomical number of microbes give rise to mutants that adapt rapidly and emerge in the form of 'superbugs'. However, microbes may have a beneficial role in maintaining the life of plants, animals and humans.

The science of microbiology has advanced from discovery of the 'little animals' in 1676 to invention of the polymerase chain reaction in 1983. Most of the microbiology laboratories in the UK are now fully equipped, providing diagnostic service in the care of patients on hospitals or in the community. In parallel with other disciplines of pathology, microbiology has established itself as a valuable support to diagnosis and treatment of infectious diseases. Major advances have been made in the fields of clinical microbiology, immunology, biotechnology and molecular microbiology; these are now part of the training in microbiology. Understanding and employing the principles of microbiology and the molecular mechanisms of pathogenesis have enabled the physician and medical scientist to control infectious diseases.

Medical microbiology offers considerable opportunities to those who want to mix clinical experience with biological inquisitiveness. The new generation of microbiology trainees has the opportunities to learn modern skills and apply these directly to the diagnosis and evaluation of the disease process. Clinical work involves a multidisciplinary approach towards understanding and solving of disease-associated problems including infection control. The latter particularly is a challenging job for those who are committed to controlling the spread of antibiotic resistance.

A trainee enters microbiology by completing training in various clinical disciplines at SHO level. Prospective candidates would find it beneficial to undertake training in clinical specialties such as general medicine, infectious diseases, paediatrics or chest medicine before joining microbiology. MRCP is advisable although not essential for undertaking microbiology training.

Higher education is in the form of four to five years' training as a specialist registrar. Trainees also have the opportunities to advance their career prospects by further education leading to a diploma in tropical medicine and hygiene (DTMH), a master's degree (MSc) or doctorate (MD or PhD) in both clinical and basic sciences and, of course, a professional qualification via the MRCPath. Recently a diploma in hospital infection control (DipHIC) has been introduced for those who are keen to take up infection control activities. The specialist registrar grade ends in the award of a CCST, which is an essential requirement for entering a consultant position.

Trainees in microbiology are also required to gain experience in virology for a period of three to six months. In addition, audits, research, surveillance activities and attending specialized training courses are part of the training programmes. Experience gained in these areas offers career prospects in fulfilment of ambitions to further the science of medical microbiology.

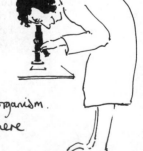

Ha! You devious little micro organism. I'd know that face anywhere

Myth	Laid-back backroom boys churning out laboratory reports whilst understanding the difference between second- and third-generation cephalosporins.
Reality	A challenging field for those who want to win the war against superbugs. The field is expanding to tackle the problem of antibiotic resistance bacteria, which have now become a political issue.
Personality	Varied ranging from highly active academic to concert pianist.
Best aspects	Mix of laboratory science with clinical skills. Excellent discipline providing training on playing with the bugs and how to solve infection problems.
Worst aspects	Isolation from the mainstream clinical opportunities.
Requirements	MRCPath

Hours

Junior   Consultant

Numbers   525 posts (five to ten per year)   33% are women

Competitiveness

Stress

On-calls

Junior   Consultant

Salary

£48 000   £52 000   £70 000

For further information
Royal College of Pathologists
2 Carlton House Terrace
London SW1Y 5AF
Tel: 020 7930 5861
Fax: 020 7321 0523
Website: www.rcpath.org

Virology

This is one of the most rapidly growing areas of clinical practice and research and also underpins many new medical diseases. The advent of antiviral agents over the past 10 years has led to a massive increase in the virology workload and the profile of the specialty. Monitoring of viral load by molecular methods to determine response to treatment is now routine as is resistance testing by detecting mutations in the viral genome. Opportunities for clinical research are enormous. In addition, moves are afoot to forge closer training links with infectious diseases. Entry is at specialist registrar level and previous experience in infectious diseases, preferably with the MRCP is an advantage. Competition for jobs is not enormous as you have to be sure you are interested in a very specific career in order to want to do virology.

Specialist registrars spend about three years training in how to run a diagnostic laboratory. During this time they learn the principles of all the diagnostic tests carried out in the laboratory and all aspects of developing quality control tests. Specialist knowledge of antiviral therapy is also acquired during this period. Clinical contact is important, mainly on a consultant basis, and often the registrar is required to advise colleagues in diagnosis, organizing appropriate tests and initiating the appropriate treatment. Most virological problems arise either in general practice or in immuno-compromised patients who provide, in themselves, an interesting specialized field of the job.

Most trainees undertake a small research project in order to familiarize themselves with laboratory techniques.

A new training scheme, leading to dual accreditation in infectious diseases and microbiology and virology, is under development with the Royal Colleges of Pathology and Physicians.

Consultant jobs are few and located either in teaching hospitals or in the Public Health Laboratory Service. Academic virology is highly competitive as non-medical scientists are also eligible for professional chairs. Virology is a fast-expanding field and there are many opportunities to be gained in other branches of medicine including the pharmaceutical industry. All in all, virology is an exciting, rapidly moving field, particularly suited to graduates who would like to spend most of their time using molecular biology and immunology in order to develop new tests and to investigate scientific and clinical problems. This specialty is small, extremely friendly and—if you are successful—provides the opportunity for interaction with clinical colleagues in the hospital and in the community as well as scientific colleagues removed from the clinical situation.

Myth	Nerds in lab coats who can't communicate with patients.
Reality	Scientific doctors with an interest in viral infectious diseases. Virologists particularly enjoy the topics of molecular biology and immunology. Clinically, they are interested in weird rashes and infectious-like diseases of unknown aetiology—could they be viral?
Personality	Friendly and approachable (virology is a small, very scientific and international specialty). An ability to communicate with all sorts from Nobel Prize winners to bewildered clinical colleagues is an advantage.
Best aspects	The opportunity to participate in some of the most exciting clinical and scientific research and development. The intellectual challenge of translating this into useful diagnostic tests and then seeing management of clinical problems improve as a result is very exciting. Learning how to recognize the most esoteric rashes can be interesting.
Worst aspects	Dealing with endless needlestick problems, signing out reams of reports, dealing with colleagues who think that virology starts and ends with 'viral titres please' and have never heard of rapid diagnosis.
Requirements	MRCPath

Hours

Junior   Consultant

Numbers   45 posts   44% are women

Competitiveness

Stress

On-calls

Junior   Consultant

Salary

£min   £av   £max
£50 000   £58 000   £62 000

For further information	**Royal College of Pathologists** 2 Carlton House Terrace London SW1Y 5AF Tel: 020 7930 5861 Fax 020 7321 0523 Website: www.rcpath.org

CHAPTER 13

Biological sciences

Anatomy

This specialty, as a medical career, has suffered in recent decades from its history, from reorganizations of medical school courses, from continuing misconceptions and from the growing discrepancy between clinical and preclinical academic pay which means that few qualified medics join its ranks. However, it should come into its own again with the increasing realization that the many cellular and biochemical details that have been unearthed need to be placed in the context of entire, interacting systems. It offers the medical graduate with an interest in both research and education the chance to pursue an interest in almost any aspect of biomedicine with a group of intelligent, like-minded colleagues, to interact with bright young students at the start of their medical course and with surgeons in training. Research topics range from conception to death, from the molecular to the gross; techniques used by anatomists often produce images of outstanding visual beauty.

The historical accident that anatomy once occupied the majority of the curriculum, combined with the pressure for a reduced factual burden in medical courses and the upsurge in new ways of imaging the living human body, means that anatomy courses have changed radically. Gone are the long hours spent dissecting small branches of nerves—modern anatomy courses are (or at least should be) in the vanguard of functional study of the living body explored by modern imaging techniques, with prepared dissections allowing an efficient acquaintance with the important basic structures. Computer-assisted learning is probably better developed in anatomy than in most other disciplines and there are huge databases of images that can be drawn on. In research, the barriers between disciplines have broken down and it now encompasses exciting advances in neuroscience, developmental biology, cell biology, genetics, biomechanics and many others. Indeed, much research is now collaborative between people with posts in different departments.

One serious consideration for any medically qualified person thinking about a career in a basic science department is the pay differential between preclinical and clinical departments, especially since the research in the two is often very similar; it now seems unlikely that, because of the pressures placed on them by the health service, practising clinicians will be able to deliver the bulk of what was the preclinical training, so staff without a serious clinical commitment will be needed for the foreseeable future. There are many compensations in an academic appointment, but money is not one of them. Anatomists don't starve, however.

Sadly, there is no recognized training scheme and very little career structure apart from the progression from lecturer to senior lecturer, to reader and, occasionally, to professor, though many senior staff and departmental heads can give good advice. A research degree (MD or PhD) and the ability to develop a line of research that is fundable in the increasingly competitive world of research grant applications, is essential for progress.

Any qualified doctor with a real interest in the scientific basis of medicine can do well in anatomy. He or she would find themselves at an immediate advantage in the teaching (and, therefore, all else being equal, in the competition for posts) as they will already have the broad background and clinical perspective required for today's medical education. Many more biological scientists without a training in human structure now hold posts in anatomy departments, which can be a big plus for research, but guard against the powers-that-be trying to pigeonhole you in gross anatomy teaching.

Myth	Academics who spend almost their entire time in a dissecting room, can draw detailed topography on the board with both hands simultaneously, whose chief interest is belittling students who can't recall all the anomalous branches of some small nerve and whose research is on similar clinically irrelevant minutiae.
Reality	Biomedical scientists from a diverse range of backgrounds involved in a wide variety of basic research, often with direct implications for clinical medicine and with a real interest in helping students appreciate the clinical and scientifically relevant element of body structure from the molecular to the gross.
Personality	Very varied
Best aspects	Success in research and getting grants, interesting and varied science and colleagues, international contacts and meetings. Lively, interested students.
Worst aspects	The long-term experiment that fails; not getting that grant; not being invited to the meeting somewhere sunny. Uninterested students.
Requirements	PhD or MD

Hours

Junior 🕐🕐🕐   Consultant/senior 🕐🕐🕐

Numbers	no proper records

Competitiveness ⚔⚔(⚔⚔⚔⚔⚔ for research grants)

Stress ☹☹☹☹☹

On-calls	none Junior none Consultant

Salary

£16000   £30 000   £50 000

For further information	**Secretary of the Anatomical Society of Great Britain & Ireland** Department of Human Anatomy and Genetics University of Oxford South Parks Road Oxford OX1 3QX Tel: 01865 272188, 272169, 272170 Fax: 01865 272420 E-mail: gillian.morriss-kay@anat.ox.ac.uk Website: www.anat.soc.org.uk

Clinical genetics

Clinical genetics is often erroneously thought of as a laboratory-based service. Most of a clinical geneticist's work involves direct contact with patients in the clinic and a sound clinical training and acquisition of counselling skills are essential.

Clinical geneticists are primarily involved in the diagnosis and management of genetic or congenital disorders, investigation of family members, risk assessment, counselling and clinically orientated research. Diagnosing extremely rare birth defects and genetic disorders and keeping up to date with the rapid advances in the subject are the main challenges of the specialty. The distressing nature of genetic disease and helping families to cope with the burden of a genetic disorder and its implications are two of the stresses.

The range of patients presenting to a clinical genetics department is very varied, since genetic disorders can occur at all ages and affect any system of the body. This gives an almost unique opportunity to work alongside almost every other specialty. There are particularly close links with paediatrics, obstetrics, oncology and neurology.

There are no SHO posts in clinical genetics; entry to the specialty is at higher medical training level. Applicants for training posts must have MRCP, MRCPCH or MRCOG. MRCPath, FRCS or MRCGP may be acceptable if accompanied by an MD in genetics. Ideally, experience should have been gained in both paediatrics and adult medicine; exposure to neurology is particularly helpful. Applicants benefit from having a degree in genetics (BSc or MSc) or having undertaken a research project in genetics or an allied subject. Gaining appropriate experience (i.e. doing an intercalated BSc and relevant postgraduate jobs) is facilitated by making an early decision to enter the specialty and planning accordingly.

The structured training programme covers clinical, laboratory and theoretical aspects of genetics. Training posts are available in all clinical genetic centres; these are located in major regional teaching centres, which are usually allied to university departments. There are excellent opportunities for research due largely to the rapid and exciting developments in molecular genetics that are defining new genes, mutations and genetic mechanisms. Trainees are encouraged to undertake research for an MD or PhD if they have not done any research previously. The number of clinical and research trainees varies from one to as many or six or seven per centre. Supraregional teaching and assessment sessions are organized because of the small size of the specialty.

Once trained, there are opportunities for subspecialization and academic careers within genetics, but competition for consultant posts is increasing. The rapid increase in demand for cancer genetic services has resulted in most newly created consultant posts requiring the applicant to undertake a substantial amount of work in this field.

Myth	Neo-Darwinians, labelling the damned from ivory towers.
Reality	An expanding and intellectually challenging specialty with a very varied clinical workload. Excellent opportunities for clinical and laboratory research. Well organized junior training.
Personality	Usually highly motivated with active research interests.
Best aspects	Highly scientific content, research opportunities, possibility of subspecialization, very little work at unsociable hours, excellent international conferences
Worst aspects	Trying to keep up to date with extremely rapid developments in gene localization and mutation detection. The distressing nature of many genetic disorders. Lack of service provision for new research development.
Requirements	MRCP, MRCOG or equivalent

Hours

Junior   Consultant

Numbers   70+ posts   5% are women

Competitiveness

Stress

On-calls

Junior   Consultant

Salary

£50 000   £55 000   £100 000

For further information

Clinical Genetics SAC
Royal College of Physicians
11 St Andrew's Place
Regent's Park
London NW1 4LE
Tel: 020 7935 1174
Fax: 020 7487 5218
Website: www.rcplondon.ac.uk

Physiology

You will probably recall meeting academic physiologists in the early part of your medical course. Physiology is the study of the function of organs and is one of the basic medical sciences on which modern medicine is founded. Life as an academic physiologist involves three main activities—research, teaching and administration—and it helps if you enjoy (or at least don't actively dislike) them all. Many universities have undergone structural changes, which have resulted in physiology departments ceasing to exist as such. However, there are still physiologists to be found, it's just that they work within larger groups such as basic medical sciences.

Research in physiology covers a huge range of studies. You might, for instance, wish to study the actions of a single type of ion channel in a particular cell membrane. At the other end of the scale you might be looking at the consequences of environmental changes on any number of functions in the intact human being. The approaches vary too; some physiologists are engaged in pure research whereas others are conducting more obviously applied research often in a field with a direct medical application. As well as designing and performing experiments, physiologists also have to learn how to present results at scientific meetings and how to write papers for publication.

Teaching involves not just lecturing but also giving practical classes, tutorials (including problem-based learning) and seminars. These require different skills, and these days most newly appointed lecturers are asked to take short staff development courses in teaching. Good teaching requires careful preparation so it takes up more than just the timetabled hours. Exactly what sort of students you will teach will vary from department to department, but you could find yourself teaching students of pure science, medicine, dentistry, veterinary science, nursing, psychology or sports sciences—in short, anyone whose course might reasonably include understanding how the body works.

Administration includes routine activities of the department (including marking your students' work), examining, refereeing papers and/or grant applications, reviewing books and perhaps later in your career involvement in the running of professional societies in the field.

Physiology can be entered at almost any stage of a university course. Medics usually come by one of two routes. Some start by intercalating a science degree during their medical course and then stay to do a PhD before returning to complete their medical training. Others come to physiology having obtained their MB BS degrees, perhaps having discovered that clinical medicine is not for them. It has to be said that there are fewer medically qualified academic physiologists than there once were; this is almost certainly due to the difference between the non-clinical and the clinical lecturer pay scales.

Myth	Nine-to-five job with long carefree summer holidays.
Reality	Longer hours, shorter holidays; opportunities to research almost any topic that appeals to you.
Personality	An inquiring mind, enthusiasm for the subject, good manual skills, interest in teaching.
Best aspects	Wide range of physiological systems to investigate, so there's something for everyone. A relatively small but good community of academics to work with. Teaching contact with bright young people.
Worst aspects	Increasing workload, increasing difficulty securing funding for research, increasing use of fixed-term contracts, decreasing purchasing power of salary.
Requirements	PhD

Hours

Junior — Consultant

Numbers around 200 posts

Competitiveness

Stress

On-calls	none	none
	Junior	Consultant

Salary

£16 000   £30 000   £35 000
with possible increase through clinical work

For further information

Physiological Society
PO Box 11319
London WC1E 7JF
Tel: 020 7631 1456
Fax: 020 7631 1462
Website: www.physoc.org

CHAPTER 14

Off the beaten track

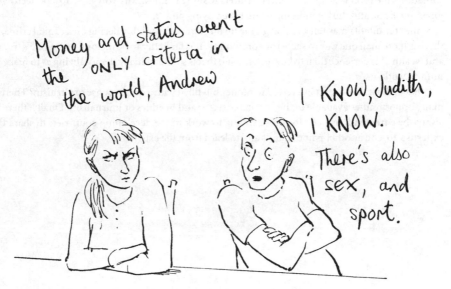

Overview

Why not escape the NHS altogether? Most doctors have looked across the fence and thought the grass looked greener on the other side. Industry offers company cars, high salaries and no more on-calls. Lawyers always appear to be oozing money from every pore and many senior doctors feel that NHS managers are paid far too much for doing far too little.

So is life better and what's on offer? The variety is simply endless. MB BS can be viewed as simply another degree and one still held in high regard. Your CV may therefore catch the eye of the bored graduate recruiter. The private sector often does pay more than the NHS in the early years, hour for hour, but remember the difference between basic salary and the hospital pay cheque including overtime and allowances. The second great myth is that the hours will be less. Although you may avoid nights on-call, the current job market is such that 12- or 13-hour days and unpaid weekend overtime are common. Sounds familiar? The last myth is that being a 'doctor' makes you irresistible; sometimes the reverse is the case with recruiters wishing to know why you gave up a perfectly good job in medicine and thus wondering if you have staying power.

Some consultants may tell you that giving up on your patients is bordering on a capital crime, but there is more than one way to serve the community. It is far better to be making use of one's training and wealth of experience than to be stuck in a job that is so individually demoralizing as to make you unfit to work.

What of those who aren't interested in money but filled with a deeper sense of altruism? There are many opportunities available in the charitable sector and in ethics or journalism. Finally, there will always be a tremendous need for those willing to work in the developing countries; to share their expertise, to lend another pair of hands and to learn from the experience.

The Civil Service

The range and scope of working in the Civil Service is so extensive that a specific job description is impossible. However, medical students and young graduates must realize that there is no training post that takes them directly into a job in the Civil Service. Thus, it is essentially a second or complementary career with opportunities for consultants of every calling and GPs who have completed their training.

For this pool of postgraduates there are possibilities for employment in many government departments, including the Department of Health, Department of Transport, the Prison Service, Home Office, Welsh Office, Northern Ireland Office, Scottish Office and Health and Safety Executive.

Much of the work means relinquishing a direct role in treating patients, except possibly within the Prison Service. The compensations are some excellent opportunities to develop and build on skills in management, administration and research and to become involved in policy formation. You are also able to move from job to job within departments to gain breadth of experience.

One of the attractions is the variety of contracts available, together with flexible working patterns which may include fixed-term contracts, secondments and part-time working. In other words, the doctor does not always have to burn any bridges to work in the Civil Service but can sometimes be seconded for an agreed period before stepping back into his or her original job if he or she so wishes.

There is a wide geographical spread of posts so that secondment to a particular job does not necessarily mean moving house to be close to Whitehall.

There is no focal point for information. The best thing to do is to keep an eye on the jobs' columns in the *BMJ* where most of the medical Civil Service jobs are advertised, or write to the chief medical officer of any of the above organizations.

Medical management and medical politics

Team practice has grown in hospital and primary care as specialization has increased, thereby requiring coordination programming and administration to cope with the complexities. Financial limitations and the training, recruitment, retention and rotation of staff all bear on the achievement of the team. Problems in these areas cannot be resolved merely by an extra effort at the time they are recognized. There is a need to look ahead, to lay out the money for equipment, devices, disposables and drugs, to meet the salary bills and reduce locum expenditure and to invest in training and development of all the professions. Long gone are the days when Sir Lancelot Spratt could opine and remonstrate imperiously twice a week and so ensure all would be well.

It was in the early 1960s that management training for consultants and the then senior registrars began in the King's Fund and the Manchester Business School. Fifteen years later every specialty had run events tailored to their own problems and five years after that questions on management were featuring at consultant appointment interviews. The last five years has seen a Masters in Business Administration appearing on CVs, usually taken part-time at a business school or the Open University. This has been the training for consultant practice, clinical directorship, medical directorship and—for a very few—chief executive of a trust.

To an extent public health medicine has been moving in parallel. Generally the specialty has focused on epidemiological technique in the identification of health need, the elucidation of patterns of disease and the efficiency and effectiveness of care. This provides a framework for purchasing healthcare, which is of vital importance to the health authorities for whom some public health doctors have become chief executives. Such work has been less prominent in the trusts who, since the separation of purchasing and providing, have rarely made a public health medicine appointment to chief executive or medical director.

The third major strand in management is the representation of colleagues on medical councils, national committees, enquiries, advisory groups, national bodies such as the GMC, and protection societies, in the British Medical Association and in regional and national education and research and development groups, to outline only the most familiar. Some might argue that representation is not management but if the success of a representative is judged by the action generated, a good knowledge of how the system works and an ability to present ideas appropriately are virtually essential. Perception, perspective, insight and foresight are all needed in developing frameworks, rule books and decision trees and arguing the case for change in a largely political arena. Hospital consultants who treat representation as an extension of off-the-cuff and intemperate coffee room remarks will find themselves out-manoeuvred.

The fourth opportunity is the political arena itself: a *sotto voce* role in the Conservative Medical Society or Socialist Medical Association or, more prominently, a role as a ministerial advisor or, for a few, as a parliamentary candidate, Member of Parliament or even Minister of Health. Decision analysis would here emphasize the difference between pay-off and utility: black pudding has a certain calorie count (the pay-off) but you'd better sell it in Manchester where its 'utility' far exceeds its popularity in London. The politician may not feel so bound by management rigour, and rely more on his touch with the people and be glad of his upbringing in the university debating society, the political clubs and the National Union of Students.

There is much to do, to suit all tastes and particularly those who field brickbats, tolerate misconstruction and remain eternally optimistic.

Myth	Neurotic bureaucrats with no concept of life at the clinical coalface.
Reality	Organizing all that is predictable in your practice to leave time to cope with the clinical emergencies and other surprises. This means your own team of doctors, nurses, therapists, scientists, technicians, secretaries and clerks but can also become your division, your hospital, your specialty or your profession. A few want to run the country as well!
Personality	Anywhere from modest integrity to Zionist zeal.
Best aspects	When your colleagues recognize your efforts gave them an opportunity. Successful development of new services and buildings and pruning as patterns of care change. Building teams and seeing the young and successful move on. Measuring success in terms of better care for patients and families.
Worst aspects	Being caught between irresistible forces and immovable objects. Watching opportunities pass by as the tired, old or obdurate hope time will not move on.
Requirements	Any higher postgraduate degree. Master of Business Administration advisable.

Hours

Juniors

Consultants
(plus time for clinical career)

Numbers	200 medical directors and 1000 clinical directors plus representative posts. About 25% women

Competitiveness

(very variable)

Stress

On-calls

(telephoned by colleagues in the evening)

Salary	Medical consultant scale with management enhancement: £50 000 to £100 000.
For further information	**British Association of Medical Managers** Barnes Hospital Kings Way Cheadle SK8 2NG Tel: 0161 474 1141 Fax: 0161 474 7167 E-mail: bamm@bamm.co.uk Website: www.bamm.co.uk

Prison healthcare

Many doctors may be in contact with the Prison Service at some point during their career but this is different from a major sessional commitment to the Prison Health Service itself or working for the Department of Health and the Home Office who organize the system in partnership. Only 225 doctors work in prisons in England and Wales of whom about 30% are female, 133 are full-time and 92 part-time. In this role they are in a position to influence the health of some of the most disadvantaged people of society: around 200,000 people each year spend some time in prison in England and Wales of which the vast majority spend a short period in custody. However all of them will come into contact with a prison doctor during this time which offers them an opportunity for a level of healthcare which may well have been absent in their lives outside prison.

Prisons are of several types including remand, local, training, high-security, young offender and open, as well as occasional specialist wings such as for sex offenders, drug addiction and psychiatric disorders. For the prison doctor the intensity and nature of the medical work varies according to the type of prison, but could be described as essentially primary care with an emphasis on psychiatry and addiction. The consultation rate is up to five times that found in general practice, reflecting the custodial environment of a prison where one of the few manoeuvres to break the monotony may be to report sick. There are also prison routines requiring the doctor to declare a prisoner fit—fit to go on a charge before the governor, fit for work or exercise, fit to be transported—as well as a general assessment of physical health and risk of suicide on admission. This assessment has to be performed within 24 hours of admission and is not easy in a local prison on a Friday night when up to 50 persons may arrive after 5 p.m. from the courts and police stations and have to be in cells in less than three hours. All this has to be achieved to standards comparable to those found in the NHS. The other aspect of the work includes the management of a hospital wing of up to 20 beds capable of sick-bay care and, in some cases, covering the needs of nearby prisons as well. Finally the prison doctor has public responsibilities for hygiene and infestation on which he or she reports to the prison governor.

A prison doctor will work within a team and liaise with the other attending clinical staff including dentists, optometrists, chiropodists, physiotherapists and pharmacists. Nursing services are provided by a combination of healthcare officers and nurses who come from an NHS training background. Social work is mainly focused in support of the courts and ultimately on the prisoner's release.

Although the prison medical officer is answerable to the governor, as a member of his management team he or she is able to make clinical decisions about the health needs of patients without interference. He or she is also a member of the prison governor's team and can influence policy in a wide range of areas within the prison to contribute to the healthy prison's culture. (The Prison Service in England and Wales is the Health in Prisons Collaborating Centre for the World Health Organization Regional Office for Europe.)

This is not work for young inexperienced doctors. Most prison doctors come from a general practice background with MRCGP or are JCPTGP accredited doctors with a special interest in mental health, or addictions or public health, and there are no juniors—the buck stops and stays with you. There are now chances for progression and the beginnings of educational development and an opportunity for a doctors to make their mark in an area where so much can be done not only in healthcare of a special group of patients but also in the context of penal reform. The salary on a sessional basis matches that of general practice and there are continual vacancies.

The special qualities expected of a doctor in the Prison Service have recently been recognized through the establishment of a diploma in prison medicine which involves a course of six modules per year over two years of which each module lasts one week on a full-time basis. The subjects include psychiatry, primary care, genitourinary medicine, audit, management, public health, occupational health, information technology and ethical and medicolegal aspects.

For further information

To enquire about the Healthcare Service of Prisoners contact:
Prison Healthcare Task Force
Room G20 Wellington House
135–159 Waterloo Road
London SE1 8UT
Tel: 020 7972 4483

For details on the Diploma in Prison Medicine contact:
Dr J Bilkhu
Course Director
Centre for Postgraduate and Continuing Medical Education
Medical School
Queen's Medical Centre
Nottingham
Tel: 0115 970 9377
E-mail: jas.bilkhu@nottingham.ac.uk

Medical research charities

The Association of Medicial Research Charities represents 104 charities whose combined expenditure on UK medical research amounted to £415 million in 1997/98. There are several hundred medical charities in Britain of which some 400 support research on a regular basis. The majority of charities fund research undertaken in universities or the NHS but a few support work in their own independent institutes or research council units.

There are two charity-sector routes which medical graduates might explore with regard to careers: a career in medical research supported by funding from a charity or a career in the medical research charity itself.

The first, a research career, is potentially varied and perhaps the easier to identify. Charities fund a wide range of research opportunities including clinical training fellowships (usually from registrar level upwards but some SHOs are supported on charity grants), which range in duration from three months to three to five years. Indeed, the Association of Medical Research Charities (AMRC) charities between them support more clinical research training fellowships than either the Medical Research Council or the NHS. The majority of these posts are at registrar level but longer-term support through to senior lecturer and professorship or consultant is also available. Clinically trained graduates often work on laboratory-based research projects and many go on to complete an MD or PhD.

In reality, a researcher is usually supported during their career from a variety of funding sources which may include university or NHS funds (e.g. the NHS regional research schemes or special trusteeships), by industry, charities or Research Council schemes. They may be funded on a personal support scheme (such as a fellowship) or might be supported as part of a team of researchers on a programme or project grant held by a senior researcher in the institution.

Charities fund a very wide range of medical specialities and encourage clinical scientists to gain experience of other disciplines and in the basic sciences. The AMRC handbook is a good source of information on funding available from its member organizations. This is published annually and is available free of charge: it is complemented by information on a website (see below). Information about other sources of funds and research opportunities is also available from the research services units in universities, NHS Regional Research and Development Directorates and the Medical Research Council.

The other potential openings are within the administration of research charities normally at a central or regional office. Opportunities in this area are hard to categorize, as all charities function slightly differently and, of course, they cover a very wide range of medical conditions and different activities from research funding, helplines, education and support.

Many medical students volunteer to work with charities during vacations to gain understanding and experience of what these organizations do. Volunteering is an enormously useful experience for all those considering a career in the charity sector, including medical graduates. Like other organizations a whole range of professional skills is needed to run a medical research charity but individuals with scientific or medical training are generally found in posts concerned with research administration (supporting the charity's grant programme) or to advise and support the charity's role in providing educational materials, information and advice to patients, their families and other professionals.

The larger the charity the more specialized the roles become. Thus, in the bigger charities research administrators may focus on a particular research programme or scientific field (e.g. fellowship programmers, cell biology or core grant schemes). In smaller charities the research officer may look after the general administration of grants and play a role in the charity's publicity, educational work or committee support.

Jobs in the charity sector will usually be advertised in the national press, particularly *The Guardian*. Specialist publications such as *Charity* and *Third Sector* are also worth consulting. There are also several recruitment agencies specializing in the charity sector. Research opportunities and scientific or medical posts may be advertised in specialist journals, such as the *BMJ*, the *Lancet*, *New Scientist* or *Nature*.

For further information	Association of Medical Research Charities 29–35 Farringdon Road London EC1M3F Tel: 020 7404 6454 Fax: 020 7404 6448 Website: www.amrc.org.uk

Medical education

Many people groan when they hear the mention of a 'medical educationist'. They assume that he or she is an ex-schoolteacher, an educational psychologist or the possessor of a BEd degree. Some are, of course; but many of the more successful ones are in fact medical graduates. Who knows better about the undergraduate medical course than someone who has been through one?

There are two routes for a medical graduate to become an educationist. Both begin by completion of the first five years of postgraduate education. Then, because there is not, at present, a CCST in medical education, it is best to get registered in a specialty (including that of general practice). Thereafter, the two pathways divide. If you want to go into full-time education, you need to get a college appointment as a lecturer. After a period in research, this would lead to a senior lectureship and perhaps, eventually, to a chair in medical education. This is a relatively rare pathway (i.e. full-time educationist); more common is a part-time appointment in medical education. Usually the route for this is through a consultancy post in a hospital, or perhaps a senior lectureship in academic general practice. Thus, you would divide your week between your specialty area and educational activities (and would be contracted accordingly).

Why do it? Medical education is currently at a crossroads. With the changing face of healthcare, the absence of long-stay patients in hospital, the recommendations of the GMC, Patients' Charters and a worldwide move towards problem-based learning, the world is your oyster. Medical colleges throughout the country are looking for help in redesigning and adjusting their courses. The opportunities for someone interested in a career in medical education have never been greater.

In the first two years after graduation, you embark on the steepest learning curve imaginable. However, the undergraduate course is failing if it does not prepare you for these first two years. Becoming a medical educationist is your chance to improve the undergraduate course and to make it a better preparation for the real world of practising medicine.

Of course, you could choose to get involved in postgraduate or continuing medical education instead. You could work in the field of vocational training or with the Royal Colleges in designing membership and fellowship courses. You could help other countries with the development of their medical courses and training programmes.

There are lots of meetings to go to all round the world. It is not just the UK which is in the midst of change. You could take a sabbatical and visit other countries to find out what's going on in the USA, Australia, the Far East, Russia or Africa. You can bring ideas back to the UK to try them out. You can take your ideas to other countries for them to try out.

Clinically qualified medial educationists are currently sought after. If you're interested in teaching and learning, why not give it a go?

Myth	Soft option: 'Those who can, do; those who can't, teach; those who can't even teach go into education'.
Reality	The only people in medical education with any real 'street cred' are the medically qualified. They've been through the whole course and know (or think they know) what was good and bad about their education.
Personality	Good interpersonal skills, persuasive, tenacious, creative, imaginative, good writing skills and sense of theatre.
Best aspects	Students love you. Medical educationists are in demand. Travel. Possibilities of high-level appointments in the academic arena.
Worst aspects	Frustrations with the system. Ignorance and lack of enthusiasm from clinicians without an educational bent. Promotion prospects weakened without strong research basis unless you (i) become dean/subdean or (ii) publish extensively in medical journals.
Requirements	MEd or ILT (Institute of Learning and Teaching) certification might help.
Hours	🕐 🕐 🕐 🕐 🕐
Numbers	There are very few full-time clinically qualified medical educationalists.
Competitiveness	🗡 🗡 🗡 🗡 🗡
Stress	☹ ☹ ☹ ☹ ☹
On-calls	none
Salary	£min £av £max
	£55000 £65 000 £100000
	(e.g. as a dean or principal)
For further information	The Association for the Study of Medical Education 12 Queen Street Edinburgh EH2 1JE Tel: 0131 225 9111 Fax: 0131 225 9444 Website: www.asme.org.uk

Medical ethics

As the advance of medical technology extends the boundaries of clinical choice, it also generates ethical and legal dilemmas. Patients who in an earlier age would have died can now be kept alive. Who should be allowed to die and when? Babies can be conceived *in vitro*. Should any woman be allowed to have a child through implantation who wants one? Through genetic screening, it will be possible for parents to exert increasing control over the physical and possibly emotional characteristics of their future children. What limits should be placed on such control and on other aspects of genetic engineering? Much modern medicine is expensive and resources are scarce. Who should get what and who should make these decisions?

Similarly, patients increasingly demand the right to self-determination in medical matters and are willing to exercise this and other rights in the courts. Many expect to be given enough information to give informed consent to treatment, to be told the truth and to exert personal control over who has access to clinical information about themselves. But how much information, truth and control can be reasonably demanded of clinicians who are often short of time and low in communication skills and energy?

The answers to these questions will not be found in clinical textbooks because they are ethical and legal in character. They focus on what should be done in relation to the patient as a person as opposed to the patient as a cluster of specific symptoms. These ethical and legal dilemmas, and risks of litigation, have become an integral component of the experience of medicine by both patients and clinicians. As result, the demand has grown for more understanding and information about the moral and legal foundations of good clinical practice, as well as associated analytical and presentational skills. This increase of interest has given rise to a host of new and exciting career prospects.

The first is, obviously, teaching. As regards medical education, the GMC has emphasized the importance of proper instruction in ethics and law. However, most medical schools in the UK still have very little curriculum time devoted to such work. This is now beginning to change and new posts will inevitably become available. The same picture holds for nursing education. Outside medicine, instruction in ethicolegal aspects of medicine also occurs in other higher education programmes, particularly the study of law, applied philosophy and social policy.

A second career path in ethics and law applied to medicine is the practice of law itself. As has already been indicated, the rates of litigation concerning accusations of medical negligence are rising and solicitors and barristers who so specialize are in increasing demand. Clinicians with legal training can also seek employment with medical protection societies which insure doctors against such accusations; however, it should be remembered that positions of this kind are rare. Even clinicians who wish to continue medical practice will benefit from legal training—with respect both to their personal legal work as expert witnesses, and to their ability to give constructive advice to colleagues and employers about ethicolegal matters.

The third career path is in journalism. Ethical and legal dilemmas and conflicts about clinical practice are rarely out of the news. All media-related organizations require a constant stream of informed writing and consultancy.

Appropriate academic training for the first and third of these activities (teaching and journalism) consists of a further degree in ethical and legal aspects of medicine, at least to master's level. There is a range of such courses throughout the UK and all consider applicants with clinical qualifications. At the institutions where these courses are offered, there is scope for further work to the level of PhD or, possibly, MD.

Most importantly, those who intend to continue their clinical careers will find that the study of ethics and law applied to medicine will increase their confidence about what constitutes good ethical and legal clinical practice. This will thus enrich their professional experience and improve their clinical practice. It will also reduce the stress and anxiety to which the lack of such confidence inevitably leads.

Law

There has always been a steady trickle of doctors retraining as lawyers. The reforms of the NHS seem to have increased the perception, particularly among younger doctors, that the grass is greener on the legal side of the fence. In reality, this is simply not true at present. The economic slump of the late 1980s and early 1990s has led to significant unemployment among newly qualified lawyers. In addition, whereas even five years ago, the medically qualified lawyer was a novelty and could use the knowledge and the experience gained as a bargaining tool in certain areas of practice, it is now by no means unusual to find yourself competing with others equally qualified both medically and legally.

A good lawyer can handle facts and apply abstract concepts to those facts. Handling and collating are tasks which clinicians perform every day. They are skills that you require as a medical student. This is what doctors do when they take a history, perform an examination, order relevant tests and then interpret the results. They apply scientific concepts to the assembled facts in order to make a differential diagnosis and formulate a treatment plan. The thought processes of doctors and lawyers, although similar, do differ in some important aspects. Whereas doctors refine their diagnosis to the correct one, lawyers, having first applied legal concepts to the facts, produce one conclusion and then go on to anticipate possible alternative conclusions (i.e. the opponent's case) and collect further facts or evidence to strengthen their own case.

In addition to the cerebral qualities that are necessary to practise law there are also qualities that are necessary in the everyday work of the lawyer. Among these are the ability to reduce complicated concepts to everyday language and then advise clients appropriately. This again is a quality that you should have gained from studying medicine. You will also need self-motivation, the ability to work alone and attention to and a liking for detail. Particularly advantageous qualities are the ability to organize your daily work and the ability to sort the urgent from the merely important. These qualities are as useful for a good doctor as they are for a good lawyer.

Assuming you wish to practise as a lawyer, you will need to qualify as a solicitor or barrister. At present, solicitors deal mainly with the preparation of a case, and barristers with the presentation of that case in court. With recent changes, however, particularly regarding the rights of audience, the difference between the two branches is rapidly disappearing.

Unfortunately, the decision of whether to be a barrister or a solicitor must be made before you start your training. You must obtain approval from the relevant professional bodies before you embark on a course of study. It is not possible to get approval from both professional bodies and then decide later. As a graduate of a UK or Irish university, you do not have to obtain a full law degree. For either branch of the profession the training consists of an academic stage followed by a vocational stage. The common starting point for non-legal graduates is the Common Professional Examination (CPE). This is an examination in six essential 'core' subjects taken at the end of a one-year full-time course at an approved institution. Information regarding these can be obtained from the Law Society of the Bar Council. Having successfully completed the CPE you then enter the legal training system at the same point as any other graduate in law.

If you want to be a solicitor you then take a further one-year examination-based Legal Practice Course. Following this you need to fulfil a two-year training contract. This is done in a firm of solicitors and consists of 'on-the-job training'. You will be paid during this training but rates of pay differ according to geographical location and the type of firm. Having completed a training contract you then emerge as a fully qualified solicitor.

A prospective barrister will, on completion of CPE, do a further one-year course of study: the Bar Vocational Course at the Inns of Court School of Law. In order to do this you have to become a member of one of the four Inns of Court and successfully negotiate the selection process for the course. In order to practise, the fledging barrister then spends a further one-year period as a 'pupil' in a set of barristers' chambers. Many, but by no means all, pupillages attract some form of award and it is usual for pupil barristers in their second six months to be able to earn fees from some of the work they do.

Competition for places at every stage is high, as are the fees for the academic stages of training in both branches. Local authority grants are virtually unobtainable, particularly for doctors who have already been through one vocational course. The obvious area of practice for the medically qualified lawyer is medical negligence litigation. Solicitors tend to act almost exclusively for either the defence or the prosecution of doctors, depending on which type of firm they work for. Medical graduates intending to become lawyers should not be too blinkered and, indeed, may wish to have nothing further to do with medicine in any shape or form. As a doctor you will have received a scientific education and obtained scientific qualifications. This background, particularly if it includes mathematics, will distinguish you from the usual arts-based legal graduate. Such advantage can be put to good use in many areas of the law as in professional negligence, commercial law, intellectual property and pharmaceutical law.

A medically qualified lawyer could also choose to become a district coroner, the officer appointed to investigate a violent or unnatural death. It is not necessary to be doubly qualified in order to be a coroner, but it certainly helps.

There are opportunities for doubly qualified practitioners acting at the interface between law and medicine, performing such functions as advising on medical aspects of a case for lawyers, advising relevant experts or acting as an introduction service to recognized experts. However, agencies providing these services are a relatively new development and it remains to be seen whether there is sufficient call for their services to sustain more than one or two companies in this field.

Finally, there are opportunities, although somewhat limited, within academic law in a university department where the interfaces between law and the various facets of healthcare delivery are proving to be fascinating areas for research and teaching.

For further information	Society of Doctors in Law and Medicine
	42 Gibson Square
	London N1 0RB
	Tel: 020 7700 7348
	Fax: 020 7700 7379

The Law Society
Information Centre
Ipsley Court
Redditch
Worcs B98 0TD
Tel: 0870 606 2555
Fax: 020 7320 5964
E-mail: info.services@lawsociety.org.uk
Website: www.lawsociety.org.uk

Medical defence organizations

In 1883 two doctors were accused of negligence in their care of a father and daughter with diphtheria; in 1884 another doctor was wrongly convicted of indecently assaulting a patient and was sent to prison. These events caused an outcry in the medical and lay press of the time, largely because the doctors had no organized professional support and no funds to pay for proper legal assistance and representation. Out of this crisis the Medical Defence Union (MDU) was born in 1885, to be followed by the Medical Protection Society in 1892 and the Medical and Dental Defence Union of Scotland in 1902. All three are mutually funded non-profit-making bodies run by members for the benefit of members (only). Contrary to popular belief, they are not insurance companies.

The defence organizations were initially somewhat introspective, much concerned with upholding the honour of the medical profession and protecting patients from 'quacks'. But the emphasis soon shifted towards indemnifying doctors against legal costs. Indemnity for damages and settlements soon followed, and the defence organizations now provide discretionary indemnity for all those medical negligence claims not covered by a doctor's employers, for example as part of the NHS Indemnity. At the MDU, a number of doctors (and other staff with a background in insurance) work in a dedicated claims handling unit looking after claims arising from private practice and general practice, with the aim of handling them as efficiently as possible.

A second but equally important function is to assist and advise the doctor who encounters other medicolegal problems which may threaten his or her interests. Help and support may be given in dealing with complaints, inquests, disciplinary proceedings (now particularly prevalent in the NHS hospital setting following the GMC's investigation of the Bristol heart surgeons and the Department of Health's emphasis on clinical governance), the GMC, criminal allegations, the police and the media. None of these issues are covered by the arrangements for NHS Indemnity. The defence organizations also provide detailed written advice (individually or through publications, and much of it pre-emptive) on the thorny medicolegal and ethical decisions which are so much part of a doctor's professional work—consent and confidentiality are the two prime examples.

With few exceptions all doctors in general practice or private practice now belong to a defence organization (essential for their discretionary indemnity for everything outside their NHS employment) and the vast majority of NHS hospital doctors do too, for indemnity and for the substantial and comprehensive advisory services. Indeed, the GMC now says that all doctors should belong to a defence organization.

A third function of a defence organization is risk management, with the aim of improving patient care and reducing or at least limiting the incidence of adverse events. Risk management is particularly strong at the MDU which has a service designed to help doctors identify, assess and reduce risks to patients and staff through an educational programme, a data collection system and a checklist-based schedule of review.

Although the ultimate decisions about granting assistance lie with Boards of Management or Councils elected by the membership, the day-to-day work of the defence organizations is carried out by teams of in-house medicolegal specialists who spend much of their time in direct contact with members by telephone (the MDU receives about 500 new calls per week) or in correspondence. They will also be out and about personally assisting and representing members at events like complaints procedures and disciplinary hearings, and lecturing on the potential pitfalls of practice, partly for education pure and simple, but also as a form of risk management and prevention. Audiences may range from medical students at one end of the scale to highly specialized national and international conferences at the other.

Any new medicolegal adviser needs a good breadth of clinical experience and expertise (and ideally a higher qualification as well) as this is essential for any organization representing so many and varied medical interests. It is unrealistic therefore for doctors to be employed by a defence organization before they have a number of jobs behind them. Even then, clinical relationships with patients must weigh heavily in the balance; time spent in general practice or dealing with live patients in the hurly-burly of an acute hospital department is invaluable.

Beyond that, medicolegal work is varied, stimulating and demanding; the additional qualities needed from staff necessarily include objectivity, analytical and communication skills and the ability to be a good team player.

Job vacancies are advertised in the main medical journals but they do not appear very often, as the total medical strength of the three UK defence organizations is less than 50 doctors; competition is therefore intense. Working hours are fairly conventional by hospital standards, but many complaints, investigations and lectures take place in the evenings, perhaps needing an overnight stay, and there is an ongoing commitment to take part in a 24-hour telephone advice rota. But, unlike clinical practice, out-of-hours work is usually planned and predictable, rather than being crisis-led. Incomers can expect to receive a starting salary roughly equivalent to that of a specialist registrar. There is a wide variety of career opportunities within each organization. Training is 'on the job', partly by planned programme and partly by interaction with colleagues. There are no training courses or individual books which can embrace all of a defence organization's activities, though some organizations sponsor their advisers on external degree courses. These are usually in law or medical ethics.

Like any other medical job, medicolegal work has its stresses and strains but those who have made the transition from clinical practice to 'doctoring the doctors' enjoy it greatly. It is a true privilege to be called on to assist one's medical colleagues in their hour of need.

For further information	The Medical Defence Union
	192 Altrincham Road
	Manchester M22 4RZ
	Tel: 0161 428 1234
	Fax: 0161 491 3301
	Website: www.the-mdu.com

The Medical Protection Society
Granary Wharf House
Leeds LS11 5PY
Tel: 0113 243 6436
Fax: 0113 241 0500
Website: www.mps.org.uk

The Medical and Dental Defence Union of Scotland
Mackintosh House
120 Blythswood Street
Glasgow G2 4EA
Tel: 0141 221 5858
Fax: 0141 228 1208
Website: www.mddus.com

Medical journalism

No one in their right mind would go into medicine with the idea of becoming a medical journalist. Most doctors do it only part-time, relying on more orthodox professional earnings for the bulk of their income. Indeed, there are only about a dozen doctors in the country who make their principal income from medical journalism, of whom two or three earn over £100 000 per annum. Most of the remainder have to work very hard to approach what they would have earned in general practice or hospital medicine.

As a qualified doctor you may have the capacity to be a medical journalist, particularly if you can write clearly and quickly (you need to be able to turn out 1000 words on almost any medical subject to order, in an hour . . . and preferably faster than that). But even if you don't have this ability there have been more opportunities for doctors who can communicate effectively to get work in television, radio, films and videos.

There is always a need for a personable 'TV doctor'. However, the fact is that only about five British medics have ever made a good living—in excess of about £60 000 a year—out of television work. But many doctors successfully make occasional appearances on TV, particularly local and cable TV. To obtain this kind of work you need to be able to demonstrate to a producer that you can improvise clear and succinct statements in a very short period of time, for instance when there are only 20 seconds left until the end of a programme! Radio work is much easier to obtain, but tends to be unpaid (or very poorly paid) employment in local radio (where funds are limited). Nevertheless a handful of doctors do have successful careers involving writing or presenting programmes for national radio. Several doctors regularly write—or even direct—medical films or videos. But many of these productions tend to be commercial, made for pharmaceutical companies and sometimes promoting a particular drug. Chances to make truly independent films and videos are uncommon.

Finding work is always difficult and nearly all young medical journalists simply have to keep applying to as many editors and programme producers as possible. The majority of applications are likely to be unsuccessful and may indeed go completely unacknowledged.

The professional organization for medical journalists cannot help you find work. Virtually all the active medical journalists in the country belong to it, but it is not possible to become a member until you are spending most of your working time in medical journalism.

Nonetheless, a number of doctors do eventually find that journalism is one of their skills and one that can be used to get a 'health message' across to literally millions of people—which is something no physician can achieve in straightforward clinical practice.

Myth	Photogenic, witty celebrities making easy money by just talking to camera or jotting down a few words.
Reality	Very hard to find work; few are truly successful. Lifelong effort to stay ahead of the game. Must be able to think and write very clearly and quickly.
Personality	Reliable and sociable. Thick-skinned. For TV you need to be very fluent and able to give concise, coherent answers very fast. For daytime TV, photogenicity helps!
Best aspects	Able to reach a target audience of millions. Fame for a few.
Worst aspects	Very poorly paid for most. Very hard to find work.
Requirements	Articulacy. Any higher qualification would help.
Hours	🕐 🕐 🕐 🕐 🕐
Numbers	about 200 about 50% women
Competitiveness	🗡 🗡 🗡 🗡 🗡
Stress	☹ ☹ ☹ ☺ ☺
On-calls	📟 📟 📟 📟 📟
Salary	£min £av £max
	£12 000 £40 000 £100 000
For further information	**Medical Journalists Association** 101 Cambridge Gardens London W10 6JE Tel: 020 8968 1614 Fax: 020 8968 7910 Email: sue4382@aol.com

Pharmaceutical physician

Pharmaceutical physicians are those registered medical practitioners who are employed within the drug industry and government regulatory authorities to provide medical input into the development, licensing, marketing and post-marketing surveillance of new and existing medicines. Physicians do a wide range of jobs in drug companies, ranging from designing research projects to getting a licence in the first place, to evaluating side effects which may spell the end of a drug's life in the last place. This calls for both general and specialist medical knowledge. Some jobs require an encyclopaedic grasp of medicine in its broadest sense while others call for the highest level of specialist knowledge about the minutiae of a particular disease. Certain skills are particularly useful, such as statistical numeracy, good writing ability and good presentation and interpersonal skills (all of which are in short supply in an industry where confidence and competence are at a premium).

There is no fixed job description, no ideal entry age for joining the drug industry and no formal career pathway. The basic job is that of 'medical advisor', and it is for advice and an inside track on medical matters that pharmaceutical physicians are employed. Most medical advisors work in the medical department of a drug company, but this may vary from a department with hundreds of staff (e.g. headquarters of a major multinational) to a department of one or two (local representative company of a multinational minnow). Clinical trials are designed, set up, run, analysed and reported by multidisciplinary teams involving medical advisors, statisticians, pharmacists and clinical research scientists of various types. The job involves liaising with hospital specialists and GPs, negotiating with ethics committees, solving problems and managing people.

Like all branches of medicine, pharmaceutical medicine has subspecialities (human pharmacology, clinical research, medical writing, regulatory affairs, pharmavigilance, pharmaco-epidemiology, medical marketing and health economics) but none of these is the sole preserve of the pharmaceutical physician. Most larger companies offer opportunities for career progression, which usually means managing more people.

Training is very much an *ad hoc* affair. There are qualifications in pharmaceutical medicine (Diploma of Pharmaceutical Medicine and Membership of the Faculty of Pharmaceutical Physicians) and companies often sponsor attendance on preparatory courses. The speciality, in the near future, is likely to be recognised for accreditation with a CCST. But for many doctors in the drug industry a Master of Business Administration is just as useful, and for those interested in the academic side of the discipline an MSc in Pharmaceutical Medicine is available as a distance learning course from the University of Surrey.

Most importantly pharmaceutical medicine is not a suitable refuge for those who do not like the demands and stresses of mainstream clinical medicine. The industrial environment is a very taxing one, in which respect is earned, not awarded automatically. Drug companies survive by succeeding in developing new medicines; they do not tolerate staff who do not give their utmost. The salaries and perks are great, but so are the demands made of those who receive them.

Myth	Glorified drug rep.
Reality	Developing new medicines for tomorrow's diseases.
Personality	Varies from the obsessional (human pharmacology, clinical trials, regulatory affairs) to the pin-striped (medical director) or extrovert (medical marketing).
Best aspects	Cutting edge of science. Involvement in developing new treatments for unsolved medical problems. Well-paid alternative to clinical medicine. International travel and company car.
Worst aspects	Administration and bureaucracy. Hire-and-fire culture. DIY career 'structure'.
Requirements	MB BS mandatory; any postgraduate membership of a fellowship, MD or PhD is an advantage.
Hours	Long and variable, including overseas travel and overnight stays
Numbers	over **600** in the UK about **40%** women
Competitiveness	🗡️ 🗡️ 🗡️ 🗡️ 🗡️
Stress	☹️ ☹️ ☹️ ☹️ ☹️
On-calls	Usually none, but some jobs involve nights spent away on business travel.
Salary	£40 000 to £100 000, plus share options and bonuses (depending on company)
For further information	**British Association of Pharmaceutical Physicians** Royal Station Court, Station Road Twyford, Reading RG10 9NF Tel: 0118 934 1943 Fax: 0118 932 0981 E-mail: liz@bapp.demon.uk
	Faculty of Pharmaceutical Medicine 1 St. Andrew's Place, Regent's Park London NW1 4LB Tel: 020 7224 0343 Fax: 020 7224 5381 E-mail: fpm@f-pharm-med.org.uk Website: www.f-pharm-med.org.uk

Complementary medicine

It is now recognized that complementary types of medicine in the right situations can dovetail usefully with conventional medicine, but if you want to be a complementary medicine practitioner, it is advisable to be as well trained as those in conventional medicine.

Certain areas of complementary medicine are more likely to be acceptable to conventional medical practitioners than others. Acupuncture, chiropractic, osteopathy, homoeopathy and hypnotherapy are the five best known. There are many other treatments which, whilst they have a place in the therapy armamentarium, have a less than secure scientific pedigree. These include aromatherapy, reflexology, herbalism and iridology to name but a few. Complementary medicine remains a fascinating area for investigation and study but is no less a minefield for that.

Acupuncture can be effective in relieving many distressing conditions, for example symptoms related to nausea, migraine, irritable bowel and hayfever, as well as the many painful conditions for which acupuncture is better known as a therapy. Acupuncture can be learned as a discipline over five years in specialized training colleges. However for the practitioner of medicine, it can be effectively grafted on with part-time training spread over some years. The scientific basis of acupuncture is becoming well established and acupuncture is very acceptable to practitioners in pain clinics and to physiotherapists, manipulators and doctors across a wide range of specialties.

In manipulative medicine chiropractic and osteopathy are best known and are the two professions that have statutory regulation. Both of these therapies require a minimum of four years' full-time study. In these therapies there is an emphasis on manual treatment including spinal manipulation to restore mobility and to improve health. Physiotherapists may also manipulate and there are many variations, including cranial osteopathy.

Hypnotherapy is gaining ground, allowing both patients and practitioners insights into the conscious and subconscious ways of thinking and illness. It is used by the medical and dental professions, psychologists, speech therapists and some other paramedical groups. Training varies from weekend courses for those already qualified in medicine or dentistry to university degrees.

In homoeopathy infinitesimally small doses of some substances ranging from herbs to poisons and minerals are used to help overcome physical, psychological or medical problems. A better understanding of homeopathy is emerging with advances in molecular sciences. Homoeopathy can be learned as a discipline outside medicine or as a postgraduate medical course.

Many therapies are now available for patients within the NHS. All of them are available in the private sector but looking through *Yellow Pages* can prove daunting. There are very few medically qualified specialists in any of these fields and becoming recognized as a specialist is extremely difficult. Most doctors prefer to incorporate a therapy within their routine practice but it is not impossible to earn a living solely in complementary private medical practice. The broader your experience in conventional medicine before embarking on a complementary therapy practice, the better able you will be to cope with the complexities of some of the problems; it is wise to have done several SHO jobs and have some general practice experience.

If you wish to make your living practising complementary medicine you will be in competition with those variably trained people in the lay sector. Working in an open market you will have to find the expertise to sell yourself and your product.

Myth	Mumbo-jumbo of ancient tradition.
Reality	Some areas are based on very good science and expanding in terms of neurology, neurophysiology and molecular sciences.
Personality	A compassionate juggler. Able to balance the patients' requests with their needs in conventional and complementary medicine and yet earn a living.
Best aspects	Hands-on medicine which is stimulating, rewarding and often fun, especially when you get results.
Worst aspects	Continuing to convince the medical profession that these therapies work and have immense value. Not achieving maximum therapeutic effects on the NHS and where these therapies are given short shrift.
Requirements	Diverse range of SHO jobs plus some general practice.
Hours	Whatever you can manage for the NHS and up to you in private practice.

Numbers

Acupuncture	Hypnotherapy	Homoeopathy
probably **2000**	about **1000**	about **1000**

(these figures apply mainly to medical practitioners with a part-time interest)

Some practitioners are now becoming interested enough to become doubly qualified in manipulation and medicine.

Competitiveness 🗡️🗡️🗡️🗡️🗡️

Stress ☹️ ☹️ ☹️ ☹️ ☹️

On-calls none

Salary

£min	£av	£max
£30 000	£45 000	£80 000 plus

For further information

British Medical Acupuncture Society
12 Marbury House
Higher Whitley
Warrington WA4 4QW
Tel: 01925 730727
Fax: 01925 730492
E-mail: bmasadmin@aol.com
Website: www.medical-acupuncture.co.uk

British Acupuncture Council
63 Jeddo Road
London W12 9HQ
Tel: 020 8735 0400
Website: www.acupuncture.org.uk

British Society of Medical and Dental Hypnosis
17 Keppel View Road
Kimberworth
Rotherham S61 2AR
Tel/Fax: 0700 0560 309
E-mail: secretary@bsmdh.org
Website: www.bsmdh.org

General Chiropractic Council
344–354 Gray's Inn Road
London WC1X 8BP
Tel: 020 7713 5155
Fax: 020 7713 5844
Email: enquiries@gcc-uk.org
Website: www.gcc-uk.org

Medical devices

This is an all-encompassing term covering everything from wheelchairs through artificial heart valves to genetically engineered human organs—in other words, everything used to treat illness or disability which comes into contact with the body but does not achieve its action by pharmacological means. It is one of the fastest growing and exciting areas of medicine. Hundreds of new biotechnology companies are springing up every year. Up to now, however, there has been relatively little demand for doctors in this industry and the number of positions advertised in the UK each year is still very small. This is changing and medical devices is likely to become a major career growth area for those with an entrepreneurial turn of mind.

There are two main reasons for this. First, throughout the world but especially in the European Union and North America, there is a move towards regulating medical devices in the same way as has for a long time been the case with drugs. Increasing litigation (e.g. breast implant cases in the USA), the complexity of many new devices and the development of new materials have dictated this, and this in turn creates a need for suitably qualified people to design and supervise appropriate clinical trials. Second, advances in such areas as tissue culture to replace, for example, joint cartilage have created huge new markets with cut-throat competition from new and established companies. In this respect, the medical devices industry is becoming increasingly like the pharmaceutical industry and this brings with it a demand for talented medical support. The difference is that the typical entrant to the pharmaceutical industry, usually with a background in general medicine or clinical pharmacology, does not necessarily possess the ideal profile for the medical devices industry.

An appropriate higher qualification such as the FRCS would be an advantage, and experience in other specialties such as anaesthetics, ophthalmology, radiology or medical physics might also be useful. Most medical device companies are relatively small although some, such as Johnson and Johnson, are giants in their own right. A doctor might be the only medically qualified person in the company and will be expected to cover a wide range of tasks from setting up clinical trials, research and development or advising on marketing strategy. The most successful may have the opportunity of entering mainstream management, opening the way to the top of some of the world's most successful companies. Doctors have a number of qualities which particularly suit them to the role of entrepreneur including intuitiveness, ability to take calculated risks and willingness to take personal responsibility for their decisions. Many of the emerging biotechnology and medical device companies have been set up by, or are managed by, doctors.

The pattern of life is different from that in hospital medicine: there is little or no on-call work but a good deal of travelling and being away from home, and the overall workload may still be very demanding. The rewards vary widely according to the size, success and stage of development of the company. A young company in the first phases of developing new products will not be in a position to offer as much as an established multinational. On the other hand, for those willing to take a risk and contribute to future success, some companies may offer part of the remuneration in the form of shares or stock options which might turn out to be very valuable in the long term.

With relatively few posts being offered in the UK at present, entry into this field may not be easy. For those interested, watching the job advertisements in the medical press and registering an interest with the established medical recruitment agencies are advised.

CHAPTER 15

Working overseas

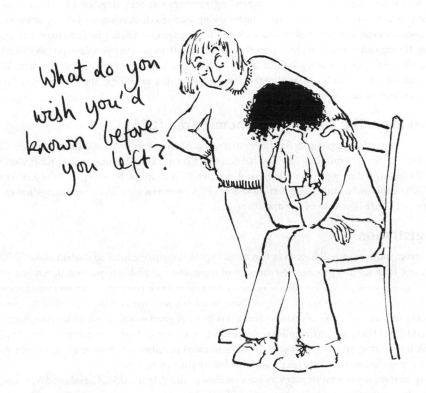

What do you wish you'd known before you left?

Overview

Working abroad can be an exciting and rewarding experience, and many doctors want to take advantage of the opportunities it provides for personal and professional growth. It could and should be regarded as an important ingredient of every doctor's training not just for clinical enrichment but for putting the NHS and one's own life into proper perspective. The options are plentiful—from development work or disaster relief with a variety of aid agencies, to specialist training in Australia or providing medical assistance on a jungle expedition. Whatever you choose, however, there will be a lot of work to do before you go and you should start as early as possible. Plan well ahead and get as much help from other people as you can.

The detailed preparations will vary depending on where you are going, what you plan to do and what you want to gain from the trip. The following sections discuss some of the most important issues to consider but there will be others. Some of the groundwork may be done for you if you are going through an agency but check nonetheless. Try to talk to as many people as possible who have been abroad themselves and ask them 'What do you wish you had known before you left?' When you contact official bodies, make sure that you get everything in writing, and keep copies of everything in case you have problems later.

Working in the European Economic Area (EEA)

There are special arrangements for the mutual recognition of medical qualifications in the EEA. If you are a citizen of a member state and have completed your basic training in a member state, you should be entitled to register in other member states. Bear in mind, however, that the process may still be lengthy and complex and that some other EEA countries have high levels of medical unemployment. There is no central registration process.

Registration

Wherever you go, you will have to be registered to practise with the local equivalent of the GMC. Be prepared for a lengthy process. The category of registration available to you will depend on where you obtained your primary qualification and what sort of work you plan to do; you may have to sit medical and/or language exams. You will have to submit your medical degree certificate (possibly the original) and will probably be asked for a certificate of good standing, which is a statement from the GMC that there are no disciplinary proceedings against you. If you are going to a non-English-speaking country, you may be asked for authenticated translations of some or all of your documents. In some cases you may need a job offer before you can register.

Registration requirements may vary even within a country. In the USA, Canada and Australia, for example, registration is regulated at regional level, although you may have to sit a national exam. How easy it is to register may well depend on how much the country concerned needs doctors; in some countries you may find it easier if you plan to work in an isolated rural post rather than in one of the major hospitals in the capital city.

Whether or not a language test is a registration requirement, you will need to have some command of the language of the country in which you are working. Even those doctors working entirely with British expatriate communities find that they need to employ local staff, refer to local hospitals, rent premises from local landlords and so on. You should also become familiar with local codes of professional conduct and practice within them, as what is considered acceptable in the UK will not necessarily be so elsewhere.

Immigration

Immigration criteria may be another major hurdle. Ask the British-based Embassy or High Commission to give you up-to-date information about the requirements. Remember that once you enter another country it may be very difficult to change your immigration status; this may affect the flexibility if you have to change your plans as you go along.

Fitting in work overseas with an NHS career

Most doctors who go abroad do so for a short time and plan to return to the NHS eventually. If you want your time abroad to count towards your specialist training, you must arrange this before you leave. The Royal Colleges cannot give credit retrospectively, regardless of how valuable you believe your experiences to have been. Under the current arrangements for specialist training it should be possible to spend time abroad, either as part of training (with prior approval) or as a temporary break within training. In either case you should discuss your plans with your postgraduate dean and keep him or her informed of your movements while you're away. If you already have an NTN when you go, the postgraduate dean will have to decide whether this number can be reserved for you while you are away.

For doctors in career-grade posts, much depends on the employer. In 1995, the NHSE circulated a letter asking regional general managers and directors to encourage the release and re-entry of staff intending to work in developing countries. Some NHS Trusts have now signed agreements with Voluntary Service Overseas (VSO), which should make it easier for staff to gain temporary release. The Royal College of General Practitioners also issued a statement in 1995 supporting overseas development and disaster relief work.

Finding a job

If you have local contacts, use them. Colleagues in the UK may also have contacts abroad whom you could approach. You will find overseas posts advertised in the classified section of the *BMJ* and other journals and on their websites, and it is also worth contacting local medical associations for details of local journals and websites.

Find out as much as possible about the job before you go. Ideally, both you and your employer should sign a contract of employment before you leave the UK. Terms and conditions of service will vary; the local medical association—which you may wish to join while you are there—will probably be the best source of advice. Also check whether your UK-based defence body or overseas employer will organize your indemnity insurance: none of the former will do so for the USA or Canada.

Remember that you may not like working abroad, so make sure that your contract contains an appropriate break clause.

Other considerations

It is impossible to give a complete list of the things to check before going abroad but some important points to remember include immunizations, medical and other insurance which you may need for the trip, schooling for your children, accommodation and transport. You must also think about the implications for your pension and how to cover your bills—mortgage, tax, insurance policies—while away from the UK.

If you are a member of the British Medical Association (BMA), its International Department can provide you with further useful information on working abroad. The BMA Superannuation Department can advise on protecting your pension rights and BMA Services can offer specialized financial services.

The red tape and preparation may seem a bit daunting but then any life outside the safe boundaries from well-ordered training programmes involves risks and extra work but huge satisfaction. If you are thinking about it then go for it. If you don't, you are likely to regret it later on in your life. If you do, you will make life-long and varied friends in the process and will always look back with a glowing sense of achievement. Employers are much more imaginative these days and an overseas experience signals enterprise and imagination and looks good on the CV.

For further information	**International Department**
	British Medical Association
	BMA House
	Tavistock Square
	London WC1H 9JP
	Tel: 020 7383 6033
	Fax: 020 7383 6644
	E-mail: snicholas@bma.org.uk

Working in overseas aid (International Health Exchange)

Doctors wanting to work in developing countries as part of the international aid sector can expect to gain experience, skills and insights unequalled in any professional training programme. Many doctors with overseas experience testify to the tremendous professional and personal benefits of the experience. Before you begin looking for a job, you need to spend some time thinking about whether aid work will suit you and whether you will suit it.

The right skills

All agencies will require a professional qualification and two years' post-qualification experience in your own field. For all health professionals this means two years from the time of your full professional registration, though if you are trying to pass yourself off as a specialist it is wise to assume that two years' experience after completion of your specialist training will be required.

Some skills and professions are more in demand overseas than others but don't be put off if you are rejected by the first organization you apply to. Different agencies employ different kinds of specialists depending on the kinds of programmes that they are operating. Some knowledge of the following subjects will also be to your advantage:

- community healthcare
- nutrition
- tropical medicine
- reproductive health
- health or hygiene promotion
- public health
- mother and child health (midwifery, obstetrics and gynaecology, paediatrics)

This list is not exhaustive and is not intended to influence your decisions about career planning or study. Nor will training in any one of these areas guarantee you a job as an aid worker. However, if you are presented with the opportunity to gain experience in one or more of these fields, then it's probably worth taking.

In addition to your professional skills, agencies are often looking for a number of 'collateral skills'. If you have good collateral skills your chances of getting a post will be greatly improved so it is definitely worth investing in your own general education. The most commonly requested collateral skills are:

- a working knowledge of language other than your own: if you speak English as a first language the most useful languages for you to learn are French, Spanish and Portuguese. If English is not your first language you should make the effort to become competent in English followed by any of these three languages. Each of these four languages is widely spoken within the aid community and is the *lingua franca* of large swathes of Africa or Latin America. Other 'transferable' languages (i.e. languages widely spoken in more than one country or region) which you may want to consider learning are Arabic, Swahili and any of the languages of the Indian subcontinent, such as Hindi, Urdu, Punjabi or Gujarati.

- management skills, particularly project management, planning, financial management, human resource management and evaluation.
- communication skills, particularly report writing, information management and facilitation skills.
- teaching or training skills.

The right qualities

While professional skills are important, aid agencies will also want to know if you have the right personal qualities for the job. There is no definitive list of characteristics that make the perfect aid worker. Indeed there is a healthy debate within the industry about what type of people should work overseas. Despite this variation, most agencies will expect their staff to be flexible, broadminded, culturally sensitive and good team players. Equally important is the ability to adapt and apply your professional training to a very different environment. Top surgeons will be of little use in rural Uganda if they require state-of-the-art equipment or a large support staff. All potential aid workers should ask themselves these questions:

- Could I work with very limited resources, both human and material?
- How would I cope in a different culture?
- Can I adapt the skills I have and apply them in a completely different context?
- Could I undertake teaching and training to share my skills?
- Would I mind doing general and administrative tasks?
- Do I have additional, non-clinical experience, such as management, that may benefit the community in which I will be working?

The right experience

Most agencies prefer to recruit people with previous overseas experience in a developing country; there is a much lower risk factor for them in doing so as these candidates are not only more experienced, but have proved that they can cope with field conditions.

Medical electives or travel experience in the developing world do not count as previous overseas experience from a recruitment point of view, so if a job advertisement asks for one year's previous overseas experience and you have done a six-month elective in India and spent six months backpacking in Thailand, it is unlikely that you will be considered.

If you come from a developing country and have spent your entire working life in such a setting this may not qualify as previous overseas experience either, unless you have experience in working in a country other than your own—for example, if you are Zambian and you have worked in Sudan. If you have worked in another developed country—for example you are Australian and you have worked in Saudi Arabia—this will not count as overseas experience for recruitment purposes.

This can be a catch-22 situation: how can you get overseas experience if no one will offer you work until you have it? Luckily a number of agencies appreciate this conundrum and will consider first-timers. Contact International Health Exchange for more information.

The right job

Jobs in the aid sector fall into two broad areas, those in emergency relief and those in development. Jobs in different areas are characterized by different working environments and terms and conditions. In addition, different kinds of jobs will be recruited for in different ways.

Relief versus development

Emergency relief work is likely to be short-term and high pressure. You might be called up with very little warning and thrust into situations that even the most experienced aid workers find stressful: famines, floods, conflicts and so on. Initially you will probably be working as part of a technical team with responsibilities for organizing some kind of service delivery to communities who have been affected by disaster. You will probably find yourself working as a member of an interdisciplinary expatriate team who generally live and work together in close quarters. Your work colleagues will be a mixture of ex-pats from your own and other relief agencies and local colleagues from among the disaster-affected people whom you are trying to assist. You will probably live in an agency compound and your personal life may be severely restricted by poor security, curfews or lack of transport. Most posts are unaccompanied, so you will be unable to take your family with you. Both voluntary and staff jobs are available, depending on the agency and your degree of experience and expertise.

Most long-term development programmes involve working in partnership with local organizations. These kinds of programme emphasize 'capacity-building', i.e. developing the skills of local people, so your workload will probably be more strategic. If your job is technically based you may be expected to train and help your local colleagues to develop planning and management solutions for their own caseload. If you are a clinician you may find yourself working with large numbers of 'paramedics' who work at community level to build up health programmes which are adapted to the particular needs of the environment in which they live. If you are working in development you could be based in a remote rural area, you could be the only expatriate in your locality or even region nd you may also be one of the very few qualified health practitioners beyond anything you have encountered; you could find yourself with very little support in the way of senior or specialized staff. You may also face bureaucratic hurdles and limited resources which make your native health service seem awash with riches. On a personal level there are unlikely to be many social or recreational facilities and you will have to adapt to a completely different pace of life. In development jobs it may be possible for your partner and family to accompany you, but you need to think carefully about their needs in terms of work and education. Again both voluntary and paid posts are available.

International Health Exchange is a charity specializing in the recruitment, training and support of health workers wishing to work in overseas aid. We provide recruitment services for over 100 international agencies working in both relief and development. We also publish *The Health Exchange* magazine and *Job Supplement*, which carry recruitment advertisements for many of our clients.

For further information	**The Recruitment Manager**
	International Health Exchange
	134 Lower Marsh
	London SE1 7AE
	Tel: 020 7620 3333
	Fax: 020 7620 2277
	E-mail: enquiries@ihe.org.uk
	Website: www.ihe.dircon.co.uk

Christian medical work overseas

Developing countries still need foreign doctors. Although many are now producing their own, the desire for higher salaries, prestigious appointments and better working conditions means that most will work in wealthier areas. Growing population, worsening poverty, rising morbidity and shrinking budgets aggravate this inequality of health service for rich and poor.

Much of the developing world's health needs are already supplied by Christian missions: in Africa alone there are over 1000 mission hospitals most of which are short-staffed. Long-termers who can learn language and culture provide a framework for those who are able to make a useful short-term contribution (usually six months to two years). There are over 20 Britain-based mission societies currently supporting medical staff abroad. Most of the latter insist, understandably, that applicants have an active Christian faith or are at least in sympathy with the overall aims of the mission. However, because most developing countries now have strong indigenous churches of their own, expatriate doctors are less likely to have Christian pastoral responsibilities on top of their medical work. The trends are towards greater specialization and team work.

Openings exist for virtually every specialty and level of training: in small rural hospitals, large teaching hospitals, public health, development work, tropical disease, disaster relief and palliative care. In general, you need at least two years' postregistration experience at SHO specialist registrar level to be useful, preferably in a combination of obstetrics and gynaecology, paediatrics, surgery and accident and emergency. In practice much training can be done 'on the job'.

A wide variety of courses are available in Britain for specific training, and support agencies supplying appropriate drugs, equipment and advice are mushrooming.

Even short-term service abroad requires careful planning, but with proper preparation can be worked into a training scheme, an established professional career or around the time of retirement. Some doctors are concerned that a period overseas will damage their long-term career prospects. However most employers look favourably on experience abroad because of the perspective, maturity, adaptability and initiative that it produces. Many eventually go on to obtain GP principal or consultant status and find that their experience has given them an edge over other candidates.

If you are married it is usually possible to find a post which enables your spouse to work as well. Also, education for children is becoming less of a problem as correspondence courses improve, especially with the advent of the Internet. Boarding schools may be necessary for those in remote locations but standards at international institutions compare favourably with the best in the UK.

This work is not for the faint-hearted and, in general, the material gains are small, but if you have a genuine desire to serve, the rewards are legion: grateful patients, a global perspective on health, first-hand knowledge of other cultures and a wealth of medical experience that cannot be gained at home. In fact, insights gained in primary healthcare, disease prevention and epidemiology, resource allocation, training of paramedics and healthcare prioritization can be invaluable in helping us see solutions to similar problems in the West.

Myth	Men in pith helmets destroying indigenous cultures and imposing Western lifestyles.
Reality	Growing need for adaptable doctors in all specialties wanting to improve health across cultural and economic divides.
Personality	A flexible attitude to cultural differences and medical technology; an interest in teaching.
Best aspects	Job satisfaction and team work; the global perspective and cross-culture experience gained; the sheer medical variety and degree of responsibility.
Worst aspects	The financial reward; the isolation (although this is changing rapidly with e-mail and the Internet); the higher risks of road travel.
Requirements	A genuine desire to serve others coupled with at least two years of postregistration experience and the willingness to learn new skills.

Hours

Junior   Consultant

Numbers	Virtually unlimited
Competitiveness	None, except for academic posts

Stress

On-calls

Junior   Consultant

Salary	Modest, but adequate to live comfortably by local standards.
For further information	**General Secretary** MMA Healthserve 106/110 Watney Street London E1W 2QE Tel: 020 7790 1336 E-mail: health157@aol.com Website: www.mmahealthserve.org.uk

Ship's doctor

Rum punches on a sun-drenched quarter-deck and formal entertaining at the doctor's table are one end of the spectrum of life as a doctor on a cruise ship such as the *QE2* or *Oriana*. The other may be agonizing over an acute abdomen or a bleeding duodenal ulcer with the nearest surgeon 2000 miles and three days away. All British ships and those of most other Flag States carrying more than 100 crew (strictly speaking, passenger numbers don't matter) are required under maritime law to carry a doctor and a limited supply of drugs and medical equipment.

There are no statutory regulations about the age, experience or qualifications of the ship's doctor: any registered practitioner will, and sometimes does, do! In practice, most reputable cruise companies (and there are some that are not reputable, so be careful) look for doctors with experience in general practice, accident and emergency, general medicine or the armed forces. The International Council of Cruise Lines (ICCL) in conjunction with the American College of Emergency Physicians has recently issued detailed guidelines which lay down minimum recommended standards for shipboard facilities and equipment and calls for doctors to be 'Board Certified' in Family Medicine, Emergency Medicine or General Medicine and to hold either Advanced Life Support certificate.

These standards are supported and met by most of the larger companies. Larger cruise ships (50 000 tons and upwards, carrying 1500 or more passengers) will generally have a medical facility with one or two doctors and two to four nurses. There will be beds for 'in' patients, limited laboratory resources, X-ray equipment and the ability to monitor and treat cardiovascular problems, up to and including the administration of thrombolytics. These ships will have limited resources to carry out surgery though in general that would be very much a last resort and most abdominal emergencies are managed conservatively for as long as possible. Smaller ships may have a sick bay little larger than a cabin with perhaps only one bed and fairly rudimentary monitoring or resuscitation equipment and very limited drug stocks.

Any doctor contemplating a career or short spell at sea must be a generalist, confident in his or her ability to cope with most eventualities, be versatile and able to think laterally. They will generally be one of the ship's senior officers in a unique position as adviser to the Master on all health matters but also as confidant to the lowliest crew member, with duties that include not only treating the sick but also entertaining passengers (the ship's doctor may have their own table in the restaurant). The ship's doctor is the only crew member in whose absence the ship may not lawfully set sail!

The rewards, other than monetary, will be the opportunity to practise the sort of comprehensive and total care that hardly exists now in the developed world but in an environment that is comfortable if not luxurious and will perhaps take one to the far corners of the earth. The ship's doctor will have the opportunity to meet, socialize with and care for people from all walks of life and of all nationalities from the very rich and famous to the members of the crew, who will often be workers from the developing world.

Terms of employment vary considerably. Some companies look for experienced doctors who will be on long-term contracts and may be earning £50000 or more, which under current UK law would be tax free while others employ more junior doctors to work alongside more senior regular employees. Such posts will pay less but can be an attractive break from an NHS career, but don't expect to have time to study for higher exams or to write a thesis, as this is a seven-day-a-week job! Others will look for doctors, usually GPs, to do single voyages from two weeks to a month, where there will be a regular nurse on board who knows the ropes and runs the medical facility. In these circumstances the doctor may be paid relatively little (about £2500 per month), but a spouse or partner may be allowed to travel free.

Jobs are often arranged by word of mouth or by direct contact with the companies operating out of the UK. A number of companies including those based overseas advertise in the *BMJ*. As always, it is important to look beyond the gloss and enquire about the details and terms of service and particularly the facilities that are provided on the ship in question.

**For further
information**   G.Waddington@Cunard

Voluntary Service Overseas

Treating malaria or snake bites may be a far cry from the usual list of a patient's ailments, but for many doctors, working at the front line of healthcare delivery in a developing country is an invaluable experience.

In Britain VSO works closely with the BMA and the Royal Colleges, encouraging the release of career-grade doctors for overseas development work. The Royal College of General Practitioners (RGCP) and the BMA have backed the drive for recognition of time spent with major aid agencies as accreditable postgraduate training. The BMA also recognizes that aid work contributes to a doctor's professional development and that the skills acquired will benefit the NHS on a doctor's return. Over 80 NHS Trusts have also agreed to grant leave of absence to staff going overseas with VSO.

Jobs are mostly based in rural district hospitals and have a varied workload, often including mother and child healthcare. Also there is often responsibility for out-based clinics or health posts, and an element of formal or informal training of local health workers. Most placements are for two years, although limited opportunities are available for shorter-term placements of 12 or 18 months.

VSO sends more voluntary health workers overseas than any other development agency in Britain. Volunteers work in 60 of the world's poorest countries, sharing their skills to help people become self-sufficient.

In addition to accommodation, a modest living allowance, return air fares and medical insurance, the VSO package also includes maintenance of NHS pension and National Insurance contributions and training to adapt specialist skills.

To apply you should have MB BS, MB ChB or MB BChR, registration with the GMC and at least three years' postregistration experience. GP training would be useful. It is important to be adaptable, resourceful and sensitive to the needs of others. VSO volunteers should be aged between 20–70 and entitled to unrestricted entry to Britain.

For further information	VSO Enquiries Unit 317 Putney Bridge Road London SW15 2PN Tel: 020 8780 7500 Fax: 020 8780 7375 E-mail: enquiry@vso.org.uk Website: www.vso.org.uk

Working with Médecins Sans Frontières (MSF): a personal view

Working with MSF is one of the most exciting things you can do as a doctor. You really don't know what you'll be faced with the following day: it could be a cholera outbreak, an earthquake or just an ordinary day of consultations; it's just so unpredictable. It's not just direct patient care. In Afghanistan, I found myself running a 60-bed hospital which involved everything from managing the cleaners, deciding where to put the septic tank, building an incinerator, ensuring a food supply for the patients and working out how to order a six-month supply of drugs, as well as all the medical work.

In the UK I work as a paediatrician and here it's unusual for a child to die. In Sri Lanka and Afghanistan the children you see most of the time are really sick and the death of a child is not a rare event. Many of the deaths are from preventable diseases such as polio, tetanus or measles. I don't think I'll ever get used to the feelings of anger and helplessness and there are moments when you just get exhausted and fed up. If you take the global view it can be very depressing. But these moments are outweighed by the times when you feel you're really making a difference, for people who are so appreciative.

What is involved?

A 'typical' MSF doctor doesn't exist, nor does a 'typical' MSF project, as both are tailored to meet the specific needs of the situation. Both the missions I've done were a little unusual in that they involved quite a bit of substitution and curative work. In Sri Lanka MSF is replacing local staff, which is something MSF generally tries not to do, but there and also in Afghanistan the healthcare systems have been destroyed by years of war, which still continues, and medical education has been disrupted.

Training local medical staff was an important component of my work. I'd never enjoyed teaching before but now I love it. Working through interpreters can really force you to be more structured and clear in the way you teach. At the same time as teaching I've learnt much from the local staff. Diseases that I'd only ever seen in textbooks before—like typhoid, cholera and brucellosis—were ones they were used to dealing with regularly.

As well as the hospital-based work our team in Afghanistan was running a feeding centre, a TB unit and a cholera-preparedness programme. We would also do basic epidemiological surveillance. So, for example, when a group of patients came in from the same village all suffering from typhoid, we visited the village, looked at the water supply there, provided some health education and carried out many consultations in the local mosque.

In the field there are no lab facilities or fancy diagnostic investigations so you just have to learn to do without. This can be hard at first and it forces you to rely more on your clinical impression of a patient—my confidence to do this has improved enormously.

Both my missions were in conflict zones where we had curfews. With MSF you usually live with the people you work with, and this constant exposure to one another, plus the curfews, plus the sheer geographical isolation can really test your patience, social skills and sense of humour! At the same time, the difficulties often bring you closer together. You have to trust and rely on each other and great friendships can develop. One of the great things about MSF is that you live and work in international teams, so you learn lots not only about the culture of the country you're working in but also about the other nationalities you work with.

What do you need?

* a minimum of two years at postregistration level (preferably with experience in obstetrics and gynaecology, accident and emergency and paediatrics);
* GMC registration;
* a diploma in tropical medicine, extensive professional experience in the tropics or work experience in infectious diseases such as TB;
* willingness to work in unstable environments;
* experience in training, supervision and management;
* travel experience in a developing country;
* fluency in English (other languages are an advantage);
* availability for at least nine months.

For further information

Médecins Sans Frontières
124–132 Clerkenwell Road
London EC1R 5DJ
Tel: 020 7713 5600
Fax: 020 7713 5004
Website: www.msf.org

CHAPTER 16

What do I do now?

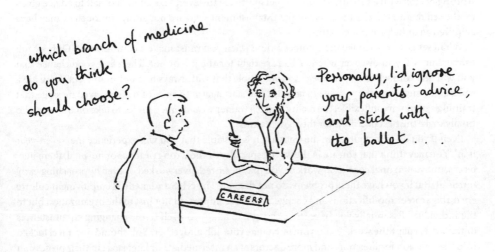

which branch of medicine
do you think I
should choose?

Personally, I'd ignore
your parents' advice,
and stick with
the ballet . . .

CAREERS

We hope that you have discovered enough about the career possibilities for you and have a good idea about the flavour of the range of jobs as well as some useful addresses. How are you going to find out for certain if the job is really for you?

Some of you may remember in the sixth form of secondary school that you or some of your friends went through a personality evaluation exercise which, on the background of your academic and non-academic interests and achievements, enabled the expert to give you some signposts about what courses and career would best suit you. It is possible that you were told you should go into theatre design or accountancy or become a restaurateur but you ignored the advice because you believed passionately at the time that you wanted to be nothing else but a doctor.

Now that you are about to be a doctor or have qualified as a doctor the same sort of career advisory services and psychometric analyses are available to help you to focus. You can talk to faculty and regional advisors, postgraduate deans and tutors, but probably the best start is to talk to your friends at medical school who know your weaknesses and strengths and who will be frank about what you shouldn't do, which is a good start. Then develop your ideas by spending time with trainees at the coalface or with young recently appointed specialists and GPs, or the young globe-trotting doctor with a broader vision and perspective. However, take a pinch of salt to advice given by the senior and hoarier members of the Establishment who are not always in touch or may have acquired an unhelpful cynical attitude.

Whatever advice you take there comes a time when you must make a commitment. Only by full immersion will you discover whether you are right for the job or not. There is a good chance that you will find yourself as a round peg in a round hole that will always fit comfortably but if you are a square peg then have the courage to admit it and start again. In spite of the perceived message that training systems are inflexible, the reality is that a trainer would much prefer to take on trainees who finally make the best decisions for the right reasons.

Even if you do find yourself in the right job it is possible that you will experience the 'seven-year itch'. You may think that you are in the wrong specialty or the wrong practice or hospital, there may be disruptive personal conflict at work or you may be bored, overworked or even approaching early burnout. But if you have these problems do not despair. The NHS and medical employment culture encourage career modifications and change, which are important not just to the organization but to the individual. Essentially you have three choices: to adapt yourself to the changing circumstances of the work; adapt the work to suit you; or change your job altogether. You should never feel locked into the same job for life: more and more doctors at an intermediate or later stage in their profession opt for another career.

Here, a specialist medical career service such as Medical Forum could help. By a detailed self and computer analysis, your various skills and interests can be balanced against your expectations to enable you to fit in with a more satisfying, balanced and achievable career goal. You may find yourself getting involved in more teaching and research, or healthcare management or charitable enterprises. You might even find yourself editing a book to guide medical graduates on medical careers. The choice is yours, so *carpe diem* and good luck!

For further information	**Medical Forum**
	Tel: 0700 079 0173
	Fax: 0702 093 3964
	Website: http://medicalforum.com

Index